And Now for the Good News . . .

And Now for the Good News . . .

TO THE FUTURE
WITH LOVE

RUBY WAX

PENGUIN LIFE

AN IMPRINT OF

PENGUIN BOOKS

PENGUIN LIFE

UK | USA | Canada | Ireland | Australia
India | New Zealand | South Africa

Penguin Life is part of the Penguin Random House group of companies
whose addresses can be found at global.penguinrandomhouse.com.

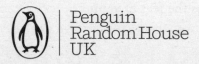

First published 2020

001

Copyright © Ruby Wax, 2020

The moral right of the author has been asserted

Set in 11.75/14.75 pt Dante MT Std
Typeset by Jouve (UK), Milton Keynes
Printed and bound in Great Britain by Clays Ltd, Elcograf S.p.A.

A CIP catalogue record for this book is available from the British Library

ISBN: 978–0–241–40064–7

www.greenpenguin.co.uk

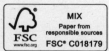

MIX
Paper from
responsible sources
FSC® C018179

Penguin Random House is committed to a
sustainable future for our business, our readers
and our planet. This book is made from Forest
Stewardship Council® certified paper.

I'd like to thank my kids, Maddy, Marina and Max, for not running away from me and Ed for not filing for divorce.

Also, I kiss the feet of Joanna Bowen, who absorbs my rantings and somehow strings them together into sentences.

Thank you to my smart and gorgeous publisher, Venetia Butterfield, and my smart and gorgeous agent, Caroline Michel.

Contents

Preface   ix

Note to Readers   xi

Introduction   1

1. Community   11
2. Business   38
3. Education   80
4. Technology   123
5. Food   157
6. World Savers   185

Conclusion   225

Acknowledgements   231

Index   237

Preface

In case you've just opened this book and are thinking, is she insane? How can she write a book about the good news when the world has faced Covid-19, the worst disaster since the Plague? Is it some kind of macabre joke or has she been in a coma? Let me explain. I began writing this in 2018 when the world was still anxious about the climate, bankers, kids' exam results, refugees and whether the 'fifty shades of grey' nail colour was still in fashion? These are still big issues but now we're facing something beyond imagination. Maybe Mother Nature has finally said, 'Enough already.' Anyway, you will notice I don't mention Covid-19 and that's because I finished this book around the time it broke; so *mea culpa*. But read on, it will give you hope when I give you the good news which is still out there.

Dear Reader,

Can I be honest? As far as fixing the world is concerned, I have no idea. I'm not an expert on fixing worlds.

I'm dyslexic so I get confused what letters stand for: IS, BLT, AA, BUPA (they're all the same to me). I usually can't tell who the good or bad guys are. Cowboys and Indians was the last time I could distinguish sides and then I rooted for the Indians – look what happened there.

When it comes to politics, economics, legislation and what the G8 summit does, I know nothing, except I do know that Davos has fantastic skiing. What I also know is that the world isn't as bad as we've been bitching about and from researching this book I've managed to find exactly where the good news lives; where green shoots of hope are peeping through the soil of civilization and may just bloom into a brighter future. My mission is to tantalize you out of the negativity zone and to paint a smiley over your doomsday face. I'm here to tell you, behind the clouds, the sun still shines.

We don't need to start packing now to go to Mars. Sorry, Mr Musk.

Love, Ruby

Introduction

You might be wondering how I can write about the future when no one knows or has ever known what it is, from the ancient soothsayers (probably reading pig entrails) to modern-day academic 'futurologists' who know jack shit.

When I say 'the future' I don't mean fifty or even twenty years from now. The future I'm talking about is your next breath. Even as I type this word, by the time I get to the end of the sentence (which I'm not at yet) that's the future. Okay, I'm at the end of the sentence, but now the future moved ahead again. You can never catch up with it, that's the only thing guaranteed – it's always in front somewhere.

My Story

So why am I writing about the future when no one really knows what's going to happen next? I was hugely disappointed when it turned out my favourite show as a child, *The Jetsons*, based on what I thought was an accurate depiction of 2010, didn't pan out. Not one thing came true: no flying cars, no robotic maids, no nothing. So I'm very cynical about futurists saying they know anything. You know where it started? It started with those old Greek soothsayers reading goat entrails. If they were legit, why didn't they know their empire was going to go kaput in a few years? And while I'm on it, why, these days, do people who claim to be psychics not clean up in Vegas? So I'm not claiming to know the future either, but I'm going to be honest with you: I decided to write on this subject because the most popular and best-selling books are about the future and I don't mind being there either.

Back to the Future

Here's the thing, you can run but you can't hide; the future is going to happen whether we like it or not, but the trick is how we handle it. Most of us don't have the courage to investigate because we're frightened to imagine change but we may as well cut ourselves some slack and be kind to ourselves. We need to accept that everything changes or we'll end up as old bores, harping on about how things used to be. We will become irrelevant, which is (alongside being unfriended on Facebook) the most frightening fate of them all.

I am aware that each of us has a different agenda: some people are just worrying about where to find food for their next meal, others are trying to cross the sea in a boat to freedom. It's only those who have the luxury of having enough to eat and know where they're sleeping tonight who can start to worry about the fact polar bears only have a few ice cubes to cling on to or that dolphins are ending up in nets.

Why the Bad News?

Why is there so much written about what's wrong with the world? I had to really hunt for positive sound bites even though they should be on the front cover of every newspaper every day of the week to replace the usual photo of a beautiful woman who is either at her film premiere or dead. Americans are addicted to the rage the guy that's President provokes (I won't speak his name because it will just make you angry), which is exactly why he's in power because when we're in a fury for a long time, we begin to think like savages. He knows how to trigger this rage and then stoke it up until we're baying for the blood of some imagined enemy. I think the more we rant, the more powerful he becomes. Every joke a comedian makes about the 'T' person gets another vote in Arkansas because they hate those white liberals and Mr T promises to help these powerless poor people. Let us not forget that this is an old technique; the moustached Mr H used it for stoking fear and look what happened next.

It's part of the human condition that we only wake up when things are frightening (see my last book); fear is what captures our attention. You might not remember your kid's first words as clearly as you do 9/11. (Those images of the collapsing towers are tattooed on our brains forever.)

We seem to be addicted to fear, getting a high on that heart-clenching, teeth-grinding, high-octane rush of terror, and when it subsides, we unconsciously look for a higher hit.

The trouble is that the fear starts inside of us and, like lighting a touch paper, spreads to everyone we know. Then people who were friends and neighbours suddenly start to blame each other for their dissatisfaction, and once they identify an enemy, *BOOM*, you have a war and a genocide sandwich to go with it. (Thank you, Mr H, for showing us how.) What frightens you then? Refugees? Ebola? China? Cyborgs? Marks & Spencer closing down? What's your poison?

A History of Self-help Books

Prehistoric Self-help

As far as we know, based on early fossil findings, there were only imprints of crustaceans; no self-help books.

1950s

At this point, self-help was targeted at women so they'd get better at being women. They were told if they wanted to please their man (and that's all most of them did for a living in those days), they needed to have a bright smile and bake him an apple pie. Wifey should greet him every night with a Martini when he came through the front door with his usual mating cry, 'Hi, honey, I'm home.' In order to pull off this happy-go-lucky domestic bliss, magazines gave you hot tips on how to be the 'hostess with the mostest' and where to score some Valium.

1960s

Now it was all about women learning to be stewardesses in the bedroom and whores in the kitchen (I may have got that wrong).

1970s

For both women and men now, the instruction was given from on high that you needed to find the real you: your inner child, your chakras, your vortex and your id. For ten long years, we searched deep inside ourselves. Some never came out; others, on high doses of LSD, leapt from rooftops thinking they were birds.

1980s

A decade where we learnt that women and men are from different planets (Venus and Mars specifically). The idea being most men are pigs and women are sheep and never the twain shall meet.

2000

That's when we went from the mind to the mouth – organic cookbooks and how to stay healthy became the 'in thing'. Yoga became mainstream and gurus in nappies made up postures involving unattainable positions like being able to give yourself an internal gynaecological exam, while doing a downward dog. Nutritionists told us to only eat turf.

2005

Spirituality became the mainstream and we were told the importance of now . . . no, now . . . no, you missed it . . . try again . . . now . . . still not now. NOW! Being in the present was de rigueur; this meant a lot of people froze to death for not acknowledging winter was coming and neglecting to get some warm clothes.

2019

Books about (you know what's coming) the future and why we should be scared shitless became number one. They were filled with words you've never met before which I will define:

- **Crispr** which I think is where you splice some genes to grow smarter kids in a petri dish

- **Blockchain** and **cybercoin** (no idea)
- **Singularity** where you wake up one morning and you're an app
- **Open sourcing** means everyone can steal your ideas
- **Robotics** they will crack the human code, suck out our brains and take over the world, leaving us as mere ashtrays

My last book, *How To Be Human*, was an instruction manual – a guide to who we are, which is a result of our evolutionary past, genes, hormones, neuronal connections, experiences, parental imprints, star signs and chakras (I threw those last two in to widen my readership). We are not our fault. The influence these have on us is below our conscious awareness, meaning shit happens and we're the last to know. So how do we take the wheel from our overworked, overstressed, overcritical minds and swerve ourselves over to a happier highway? We have to drastically change our old navigation systems that drive us to despair, to a more positive destination. If we don't, we'll forever be breaking down. There is no AA service coming to help us. It's up to us.

We need to learn to pull over and calmly look inside the bonnet (I mean our minds for those of you who don't get metaphors).

If we could treat ourselves with more compassion, realizing that our glitches are not *our* condition, but the human condition, we just might be able to change ourselves for the better and that would ripple out to the world. I've said it before: we work like neural Wi-Fi. We have the equipment in our brains to make some internal adjustments, train our brains to be kind, not cruel, and if we do, the future is bright. If someone hurts me, I want to hurt them back. If I envy someone, I want to steal what they've got. But on the optimistic side, if someone cares about me, I'll care right back. That's how we roll as individuals and as a society. I'm picturing us as a long line of dominoes and the first in the queue knocks over the next, each sending the message of empathy and compassion.

Good News

At this time things are better than at any point in history unless you believe in Camelot.

Life expectancy, they point out, has risen more steeply in the past fifty years than the previous thousand: a child born in 2016 stands a fairly good chance of seeing the arrival of the twenty-second century.

In the last couple of hundred years, from a world that was almost completely illiterate, 84 per cent of adults have learnt to read.

In 1981, almost half the people in the developing world lived below the poverty line; as of 2012, that figure had dropped to 12.7 per cent.

And most surprising of all . . . The last decade was the most peaceful in the history of the world. Yes, it turns out that being around in the Spanish Inquisition was slightly more stressful than Brexit. At least you're not going to end up with a spike through your head . . . yet.

What I Do Know

From the research I did for my last book, I think I have more of an understanding of why we think, act and feel the way we do. I've studied my own mind as a microcosm of the human condition and put it under a microscope to observe my inner monologues. Let me tell you, it's a shit show of regrets, incrimination, revenge, envy . . . But by practising mindfulness, I've learnt, it's better to be aware of what's going on in your mind. If you aren't, you'll project your poison on to other people and then blame them for your own flaws. What we think to ourselves is how we treat other people, but knowing that we all have similar thoughts running through our minds (same recordings, different lyrics) has made me far more tolerant of people because we all have the same surround-sound, just with slightly different themes and in a variety of languages. 'I'm an asshole' packs the same punch in Spanish as in Mandarin.

There should be an app where people admit what's really going on in their lives; 140 characters on our low self-esteem. It could be called 'Shitter' instead of Twitter. You'd probably become incredibly popular and get millions of followers because the rest of the world would identify. Let's all agree that the happier people look on Instagram photos, the more miserable they probably are inside. You can often equate smile size with levels of internal mayhem. And these days it's not throwing spears or missiles, it's trolling that's our modern-day weapon of mass destruction.

Compassion

On rereading my last book – something I rarely do because I immediately start doing corrections in spite of the fact that it's too late, the book's already been published – anyway, since then, I've realized that maybe in some areas I came to the wrong conclusions. (Very few authors will admit they were wrong; I think it shows humility and a youthfully flexible mind.) Instead of my theory that we're born vicious with a 'dog-eat-dog' mindset (though personally I've never seen a dog eat a dog), I've come to the conclusion that we're born with a more compassionate nature; we've all got this thing called compassion dust, it's just that some of us don't know how to sprinkle it.

I used to call it the 'C' word; I was very queasy saying the word 'compassion' (see, now I can say it) but recently I've discovered it's the most crucial thing to have if we want a good life. You can read as many books as you like on how to be a big-deal, powerful leader who commands his team like a general but power will never give you that warm, wind-chimey feeling of calm. You may get a yacht, a private jet and partner with no wrinkles, but you'll be unable to feel real joy.

Here's the Hope of the Future

Do you think it's possible we would fare better in the future if we were kinder to ourselves and everyone else around us? Would that bring in the good news? We're experts at revelling in the bad stuff, but now we'll have to focus more on compassion to improve ourselves as humans. Paul Gilbert, creator of mindfulness-based compassion therapy, says, 'Developing compassion is like playing a musical instrument – it's a skill that can be enhanced with dedicated practice.'

Nothing will change until we change the lens through which we see the world. As Albert Einstein said, 'We can't solve the problems we face with the same thinking we used to create them.' My mission in writing this book is to find out where the green shoots of hope are and who is tending them.

It turns out there is a new world view waiting in the wings to replace the old one. The examples I give in this book of inspiring innovations and innovators in education, tech, business, community and food will make you more hopeful about what's on the horizon.

I'm also hoping the experiences I'll have, places I'll go and people I'll meet will inspire me to change my life in some way. I'm beginning to realize that, unconsciously, I clearly wanted to make a change and writing this book was partly an excuse for me to discover what that is.

By the end, will I be enlightened? More compassionate? More confused? The same as I am now? I just cross my fingers I don't go AWOL, give away all my money, go off-grid and live with gorillas.

You might not be surprised to learn that the first chapter is about building community as an antidote to loneliness. If our natural state is working together and caring for each other, we need to find community and rethink how we can live together to treat one another with care and respect. Enough with the intro, let's move on.

1

Community

The biggest cause of suffering these days is not, as some of you might think, panicking about finishing your 10,000 steps because some wristband barks at you to keep going, even after collapsing. (I always wonder how many people die of strokes because they only did 9,999, lying there on the ground, their little legs still kicking to finish that last step before they croak.) No, the biggest cause of emotional pain in the Western world is loneliness. This feeling of isolation is the main cause of the decline in mental health, which has a direct impact on physical health. It's like your body is a pinball machine: once the ball of stress shoots out from the flippers, it takes out your immune system and then you're a welcome mat for the diseases that can kill you. Loneliness is not just some lightweight Elvis song that twangs the heartache of being left out, it is activated in the same part of the brain as physical injury; being side-swiped on Tinder hurts as much as snapping your femur. It probably feels worse, because with a broken leg you might think, 'I'm such a klutz,' which is far kinder than thinking, 'I'm a loser, everybody hates me.' Research now shows that people who are isolated, on average, have shorter lifespans than those who have a solid social network. The sense of isolation is so agonizing that they say prisoners prefer to have violence inflicted on them over being sent to solitary confinement. So even though we think we want privacy, what we really need is other people.

Why Are We So Lonely?

We are the first species in two million years to disband its own tribes. Families disperse, neighbours hardly know each other and, even though we're supposed to be the smartest beings on earth, we've lost the plot; we've lost the point of us and it turns out that the point of us is to mingle.*

Robin Dunbar, the evolutionary psychologist, points out that if you are an influencer you could potentially have 5 million friends but still may be the loneliest person of all, having to paint on your own reflection day and night in order to convince the rest of the world you matter. I saw a documentary where a terrified Paris Hilton jack-knifed up from bed each morning, clawing for her phone like it was a syringeful of meth to see if she'd lost any of her 50 million followers while she was sleeping. She was convinced she had such a close affinity to them all. Throughout her day, she watched her ratings like a trader watches his stocks, her self-esteem zigzagging from narcissistic rapture to thoughts of suicide.

Luckily, most of us on the planet still know what it feels like to have a close friend. We 'feel seen' in their presence and they see us in all our heiniosity and they still love us. (I made that word up for anyone trying to look it up.) This feeling of 'being seen' is now mistaken for being seen on a screen and that is not what I'm talking about. You can only 'feel seen' in the flesh because it's not your looks that evoke emotions (except for the very shallow), it's the vibe two people create together, or to be more scientific, it's the hormones

---

* Now, as I reread this in lockdown, that seems so poignant.

you both spurt at each other. When someone makes us feel good and safe, we manufacture oxytocin in our brain and this in turn switches on the mechanism in their brain to brew up their own stash of oxytocin – so now you're getting high together. If we feel good, people will like us, and the more people like us, the better we feel. Nature really knows how to make a win-win situation work. The oxytocin doesn't just induce feelings of pleasure, it stimulates empathy and compassion, which are also contagious, and so we infect each other with kindness and that is when the human race is at its finest.

Conversely, when someone doesn't like me, I can sometimes smell it. In the past, if I picked up that whiff of a sneer, I'd turn myself inside out to get their approval, attempting to be hilarious, which always backfires because they can smell your desperation too. Nowadays, though, if the hate-smell is strong, I just retreat because I have learnt that how someone sees you is really none of your business; it's the film they're playing of you, nothing to do with you, so move away from the building.

Connection From Birth

You can run, you can hide, but it's in your DNA to connect. Henry Thoreau was one in a million in being able to live alone on Walden Pond out in the woods for years; the other 999,999 people who attempt it would go nuts in all that isolation and end up gnawing their own legs off.

It's perfectly simple, we all want to be happy so we hunt for others who can press our 'happy button'; this is why comedians have jobs. When they make someone laugh, they're only really switching on their audiences' endorphins and, even better, charging money for doing it. They make them pay for something the listeners are manufacturing in their own brain; comedians are just fluffers, turning on everyone's happy juices. And that feeling of shared exhilaration spreads like wildfire through the room. The bursting feeling of bonding happens when people understand the same joke. Then they feel connected, stress levels lower and the oxytocin flows, making them feel like they're all tucked up safe and sound, sucking their collective thumb. When we laugh together, it implicitly means we see the world the same way and that's when we go into bond mode. Words and actions can be misinterpreted, but laughter signals pure unadulterated mutual recognition. Cows moo to find each other, sheep bah, horses neigh. Humans laugh. This is how we recognize our tribe. (Boohoo is also a globally identifiable noise but it's not so much fun and people don't like you for passing it on to them.)

My Story

I remember once going to a Born Again Evangelical meeting. (I wish I believed in Jesus, so many of my problems would be solved.) You go into those churches and everyone's clapping and singing unashamedly, heads thrown back, uvulas flapping. You can and are encouraged to hug your neighbour without being hash-tagged as a pervert. You actually have to 'love thy neighbour' because those are the rules. Nobody minded there that Jesus and I weren't on first-name terms. God bless him, the priest took my hand and led me to the front, put his hand on my head and threw me into the arms of two 'brothers', while whispering in my ear how to talk in tongues. (Basically, you foam a lot while blithering.) I'm telling you, I felt wrapped in a duvet of love. It was like my body was filled up with some warm liquid or like I'd swallowed a purring cat. For a moment. Then, when I left, I felt only envy for their united faith in 'Him' while I, the imposter, skulked off to my isolation where I continued to hunt for my tribe. Guess who's happier? Me or the believers? Duh!

Linking Brains

About 100,000 years ago, our brains increased to three times their original size. Neurons suddenly started to connect at a crazy pace, like trees sprouting branches in fast motion. This larger brain didn't evolve to give us the ability to beat the competition as is believed. We grew more neural connections to make more social connections and a strong network ensures survival. If no one has your back, you might as well be dead meat. So, the more neural connections, the longer the contact list.

This increased brain size gave us more advanced ways of playing with and supporting each other. It's not just that we socialize in order to live, it turns out that we live in order to socialize.

But another part of our human condition, which is a bitch, is that we're pulled between wanting to be in with the crowd and wanting to be alone, as Greta Garbo kept saying, and boy, did they leave her alone in the end.

My Story

This is the quandary that can tear us apart throughout our lives and I know this in my deepest bowels; if I'm not invited to a party I feel bereft, and if I am, I'm even more miserable, knowing that I'll have to jerk myself into a rictus of hilarity to seem interesting and therefore be invited to more parties . . . which I'll hate.

Even the words 'drinks party' freeze my blood. There's that sick-making moment when you enter the 'drinks party' room and everyone seems so adult, chuckling in relaxed clusters, holding their glass of 'bubbly' (I hate that word even more). I'm in a sweat, dizzy with anxiety over who to approach; scanning like a buzzard for who looks interesting and who, if anyone, might be interested in me (I mean the real me, not the one who improvises her schtick on the spot, to amuse and cover the fear that someone might suss she's not that smart or, worst of all worsts, that she's boring). Why does it always feel like I'm auditioning to play the part of someone scintillating and why does it matter so much that someone I'll never see again or who I don't give a shit about, likes me? Like dancers, the rest of the party people seem to know when to move to a new partner or remain chit-chatting to the person they're facing. They seem to know when to turn and move away gracefully. I have not received the choreography notes so I just stand like a startled skunk before you run it over while someone spews at me a full report on their child's grades in face-painting (I think their kid is twenty-five).

But one thing we do have in common is that we're all judging each other within seconds of a sighting. I instantly start sniffing out whether I'm smarter, more successful or more talented than they are and they're doing it right back at me. All the while you're getting 'in-coming', subtle feedback on where you are on the totem pole of popularity. You can tell how you're doing by the flicking of eyes away from your face in mid-sentence, indicating you're dead ... you may splutter a few more witticisms, but you're fried, they've spotted a higher being over your shoulder.

The lesson here is, stay at home ... but then you're alone and start having that 'no one likes me' kick in the heart. I don't know which is worse, suffering the pain of isolation or having to listen to someone's views on Brexit. Both make you want to kill yourself.

Frazzled Cafes

This is exactly why I started my charity called Frazzled Cafes. I wanted to create a safe place where small groups of people could meet and speak honestly to each other without the fear of appearing weak. My belief is that being vulnerable isn't being weak, it's being human. I created these cafes for people I described as 'frazzled', which isn't a mental illness, it's just the state most of us find ourselves in when our lives got faster than we could live them and so we went into a tailspin. I thought, why not find a group of like-minded people who also want to find where the ground is? A meeting place where we could cut the cocktail crap and talk straight from the heart. This mode of communication isn't mutual moaning, nor is it delivered in po-faced seriousness (I'm often at my funniest when I'm most honest), it's where we mutually abide by the rules of authenticity. It's not therapy or self-help, it's more like a club where you have to go as close as you can to being genuine. When I go to a Frazzled Cafe meeting and listen to people spill their lives, with no frills, I leave feeling liberated from my feeling of isolation. No theatre, concert or lecture can ever give me that same feeling of elation as when a meeting is over and we all feel that universal bond, like our hearts are all chained together on the human charm bracelet.

These people are strangers when I walk in but each time I leave, I love them because they were brave enough to show me a little piece of who they are. If you want to come to a meeting in one of the many cafes up and down the UK, please sign up on FrazzledCafe.Org.

I'm aware that in every city, town and village there's an endless stream of groups where you can meet people with similar interests: pot-throwers, foodies, the over-sixties, young mothers, over-eaters, volunteers, clubs for everything, including groups who like to have sponges thrown at them, educational courses and, let us not forget (even though the numbers are dwindling), churches, synagogues, Buddhist centres, mosques and so on . . . These all create community because of shared interests or being with people who are like you. Please don't think I'm overlooking meetings where people have a common mission to help in areas where the system has failed; Extinction Rebellion, Help the Aged, soup kitchens and food banks, etc. (I will cover some of them in the last chapter, titled 'World Savers'.) What I'm talking about in this chapter is the kind of community where we're not bound by our similarity, but one where diversity is valued because the members have recognized each other's sameness. If you peel back anyone's skin (please not literally) you'll find someone just like you and that is when the world loses its terror and we all become the human race.

I realize these types of 'honest talk' get-togethers are not for everyone; some people may actually prefer swigging poison to joining that kind of group, but it's what I'm after (and it's my book). Maybe if I'd had an extended family who loved and supported me whatever I did and we'd all spent Christmases together laughing around the tree, I wouldn't feel the need to find that kind of compassionate community, but I didn't, so this, for me, is the next best thing.

My Story

Whenever I used to watch those animal docs, I always identified with that lonely elephant who strayed from the herd, lost forever, until they keeled over in the dust. I knew what that felt like. When I was young, I lived across the street from a public park and watched families and groups of friends having picnics; old and young, laughing together as they barbecued chicken and ladled out the slaw. I was smothered in envy, sitting in the picture window next to my dog, who also wanted out (though his ambitions were slightly different to mine; he just wanted someone to hump and my mother refused to let him out unless he was connected to a leash). I wouldn't even have needed a chicken leg, I just wanted to be in their barbecued warmth. Maybe in real life those happy families hated each other, but from my POV, it was the American dream. This yearning could have been because I was an only child and felt I needed a larger group of people to protect me from my unhinged parents whose idea of child-rearing involved using a belt for 'teaching me a lesson'. My short-fused father once chased me across the street while trying to smack me for some misdemeanour. I ran into a random house and instinctively the family formed a circle to protect me from a wildly flailing and shouting daddy. This could be why I'm always looking for this kind of igloo of human warmth to protect me from potential danger.

Another place I found salvation was at a summer camp called Agawak, meaning dead Native American or something. The only reason I'm sane (though some would argue) is because my parents sent me each year to the North Woods in Minocqua, Wisconsin, among the evergreens and lakes, where we campers, free of the oppression of ambitious parents, lived in log cabins.

Free at last! I can still sing, much to my friends' distress, 447 camp songs. (If I'm drunk, I try to sing all of them at parties. For example – this following song is sung to the tune of 'Smoke Gets in your Eyes' – '*When camping days are through, we'll remember you, blue team. The friendship and the trust have always been a must, I'll always be true . . . to you.*' I'm weeping now as I'm typing this.) On day one of camp you're assigned to a team, either blue or white. To this day I will take a bullet for any fellow blue. Back in the day, we would pummel the white team in life-or-death canoe races, using our paddles as weapons. I went to camp for eight glorious years and at the end of my time there, my parents had to drag me out by the ankles, my nails deeply embedded in a totem pole. Ever since, I've been looking for a replacement for the blue team.

Then when I had kids, I was in dire need of a tribe. It's probably a primal pull-back to the old Homo erectus days about 400,000 years ago when I was young and all us new mothers shared childcare around the fire, our dangling breasts available to anyone who needed filling up like human petrol pumps. So when I became 'a mother', I, more than anyone else I've ever known, needed other mummies to help me, as I was useless at basics like which side up do you lie the baby when changing nappies? I did find other mothers to help me and some I'm still friends with and love. There were others, however, who were bores, always yabbering on about how engorged their cervix was on delivery. I had nothing to contribute as I had been on drugs when I gave birth and had no memory of the event. I remember one mother at a coffee morning holding forth on what a disgrace it was that someone's dog was excreting in the communal gardens. She called it her 'anti-poo' campaign where she put little flags in the dog stuff that said, 'Whose is this? Would you like me to do this on your lawn?' (I swear this is true.) And she wanted me to join her vigilante team.

A few years ago, I had the idea (I didn't tell Ed, my husband) that I would invite hand-picked people to live in my house, creating a community at home. The kids had abandoned me when they left home, so screw them, I decided to find replacements. I got my first inmate, Thubten, the monk who eventually helped with my last book and who toured the subsequent show with me. I had heard him speak at a conference and immediately asked if he'd like to live in my house whenever he was in the UK. (Thubten is a mindfulness teacher/globetrotter, from Google to universities to the UN.) I've given him a little monastery he can call his own at the top of the house. So when he's in town, he comes down the stairs in full robes and either we meditate together or he makes me laugh with his outrageousness. I tell everyone I invited him to live with me because he matches my sofa but it's really because he gives great lines, which I steal. I also use him to return things that I've bought when I don't have the receipt. He can go into any shop because no one would think a monk would pull a fast one.

Also in my search for community, my friend and editor of this book, Joanna Bowen, rented me a shed on her farm, which I turned into my Nano house.

(Nano is a tiny one-room building for smaller living.) In mine, I sit at my desk in front of a large window facing cows and fields. She lives in the big house with her enormous family and a non-stop stream of interesting people. I've met graduates who grow artificial meat, architects, newspaper editors, authors, actors, farmers, chemists, and once Prince Harry walked through the kitchen, I do not know why. I even met my neuroscientist friend, Ash Ranpura, there, who along with the monk, helped write my last book and also toured in my show. He too now sometimes stays in my London house. Anyway, when I go to the Nano, I can walk thirty feet to Joanna's house to communally eat with fascinating people or stay in the Nano where there's nothing but silence and cows.

Future Communities

I am just reminding you all, including myself, that this book is about the good news and this chapter is supposed to talk about how we'll live in the future. I keep finding books and articles which seem to spread dread of even more isolation, which the doomsday soothsayers predict because of rising populations that are inevitably heading for a soulless dystopia of high-rise hell. Even now you can see those towers are being ghettoized, cut off by spaghetti-looping motorways. High-rise islands of offices, living spaces, restaurants, supermarkets, shops, nail bars (God forbid there are no nail bars. You may be a mental wreck or the size of Bolivia but as long as your tips are coloured everything is fine), so you never have to leave your walled city. To me, these clustered, entombed glass-and-steel fortresses all look the same as each other, with the same branded shops. The inhabitants will no doubt also go the way of Gap, all becoming identical.

We are told that people prefer anonymity to limit the Big Brother-type surveillance; the walls, the forks, your fridge is spying on you as we speak. The trouble is, yes, you can have your privacy, but what about social ties? No longer can you borrow that cup of sugar from the neighbour; they probably won't even unlock their door for you, fearing you might rob the place or take the dog as a hostage. In the old days, if you needed a plumber, a babysitter or a shoulder to cry on, there was usually someone in your building who had those skills or at least could suggest someone they knew to help. Now, we have to call agencies to get someone over and then pay through the nose for their services.

But rather than live in teeth-chattering fear about what's here and what could be coming, let me steer your attention to the hopeful signs that might point to an exciting future. So, what's on the horizon and what are the more enlightened city planners and architects working on now?

Urban Planning: *The Good News*

We've only lived in cities for the last 6,000 years so we're in the foothills of what works to make a more human-centric neighbourhood. Previous developers had no idea what they were doing; one monster building, almost touching the clouds, is at arm's length to the next and the next to the next . . . They can watch their neighbours' television through the window but will probably never make eye contact with them.

But now planners have woken up and come to the conclusion that we need to create developments which help us live together rather than sitting in separate pools of loneliness, once in a while sending out tweets like ships sending out flares to say they're sinking. They've realized that the designs of cities aren't actually conducive to human beings who might want to make contact with other human beings and that blocks of flats surrounded by empty communal spaces don't work as well as closely spaced housing with wiggly paths connecting them to encourage people to mingle.

Julian Agyeman, an urban planner, thinks that the future of humanity is going to be mostly urban and that spaces should encourage the sharing of resources. In his book *Sharing Cities* (co-authored with Duncan McLaren), he proposes a new 'sharing paradigm', encouraging trust, connection and collaboration. Case studies of various city projects show how sharing could 'shift values and norms, encourage civic engagement and political activism, and rebuild a mutually collaborative support system'.

One of the case studies in his book is on the city of Copenhagen. The Danes have not always been keen sharers but as the famous urban designer Jan Gehl says, 'People of any culture are the same the world over. They will gather in public if you give them the space to do it.' Copenhagen is encouraging people to spend a longer time in its public spaces so that they are less focused on their destination and enjoy the journey. So the street architecture (benches and planters) are supplemented with brightly coloured adult-sized hammocks made from recycled fire hoses luring you to lounge, swing and linger. Seventy-five per cent of buildings have glass walls on the ground floor to make it possible to see in and out. (I love nothing better than being able to see into people's homes although they don't like it as much as I do.)

One of the sites is in the most ethnically diverse area, Nørrebro, a park designed to 'reflect diversity' by filling it with artefacts and structures from fifty different cultures;

you can gather on Iraqi swings or Brazilian benches around a Moroccan fountain under Japanese cherry trees while eating international cuisine. You'll never have to travel again.

There's also the most developed cycle network in Europe with cycle paths running between the parked cars and the kerb so that the parking becomes a barrier between the bikes and traffic. (If you get out on the passenger side of your car you can score a home run by sending the cyclist flying into the outfield.)

The City of Cyclists hopes to be the world's first carbon neutral city by 2025 and in 2014 was awarded the European Green City Award.

Living Cities

'Living cities' have started to sprout in places like Singapore where the government subsidizes green buildings. They grow plants and shrubs like sideways forests all over the walls of skyscrapers, called 'vertical gardens'. (Mowing them may prove hazardous.) This cools the buildings, absorbs carbon dioxide and attracts wildlife which may otherwise be dying out. Imagine looking out of your window and seeing a beaver climbing up your wall. Who do you call?

Also, in these cities they're encouraging 'green roofs' where a garden is built on the fortieth floor or beyond. The trouble is, unless you're building from scratch, how do you convert a huge city to a non-carbon one? If you're in China, there's no problem, you just announce you want a zero-carbon mega city on pain of imprisonment and, boom, it's up within hours.

Another project in Asia is led by an architect called Kengo Kuma, working in Tokyo, who says, 'I want to reshape the city. I want to break space up and return things to a smaller scale.' This includes planning for more trees and parks; places where people can make connections with one another. Tokyo had to develop very quickly after the war which is why it grew in such a haphazard and squashed way, leading to a syndrome called *kodoshi*, meaning the lonely death. He goes on to say, 'My students all live in shared housing now. That's new; we've been living in isolated spaces, separated by concrete. People don't want to do that any more.' He also wants to create village-sized communities. I say good luck to him, in a population of 126.8 million he'll have to build them in the sky. (And they'll have to find space for all those waving plastic cats and terrifying dolls with giant eyes. They have rights too.)

Non-tech Solutions to Urban Living

Julia Watson, a lecturer in urban design at Harvard and Columbia Universities, has suggested really interesting non-tech solutions to keeping cool without relying on air con, which is one of the biggest contributors to carbon emission. Covering the rooftops in trees and plants can cool a building by 60 per cent. She says the high-tech ideas for cities are born out of 'the same human superiority-complex that thinks nature should be controlled'. Instead of trying to be smart, she suggests ways to be dumb and just let nature do its thing without interfering too much. You can grill a pork chop or sunbathe on a lounger while the greenery helps suck up rainwater, lowering the risk of flooding, helping reduce air pollution and greenhouse gas emissions . . . but I have vertigo so I won't be living there.

Floating Cities

I love this idea. In Asia, about 3 million people move from the countryside into cities each week, and the majority are heading towards coastal cities which now contain over half the world's population. The UN Habitat prediction is that by 2035, 90 per cent of all megacities (over 10 million people) will be on the coast. So a solution being floated by the UN is 'floating cities'. Oceanix City, or the world's first sustainable floating city, will consist of groups of hexagonal platforms, anchored to the seabed, that could each house around 300 people, effectively creating a community for 10,000 residents. Cages under the city could harvest scallops, kelp or other forms of seafood. Marc Collins Chen, the chief executive of Oceanix, says the technology to build large floating infrastructure or housing already exists.

I'm picturing a scenario where, in the future, if you want to go on holiday, you simply up anchor and move to the destination of your choice; the problem would be that the whole neighbourhood has to come too.

BedZED Eco-community

Closer to home, in London, there's an eco-community called BedZED that's now twenty-five years old. In the middle of a normal-looking South London street, there's a very cool living complex where they have no heating bills, solar panels, green spaces, a large allotment for growing your own vegetables and a communal space where you can learn yoga, karate, cooking, dancing and drink and have coffee. I almost turned around to pack my bags and move in. This complex is owned by the Peabody Trust, a housing association which has moved with the times and alongside BedZED acknowledges that 'poorer people are in the section of society that will suffer first and foremost if we do not find a more sustainable way of life'. So BedZED has become a test bed for developers and builders to learn about the future of housing, particularly social housing.

Hundreds of residents live in the two-storey, glass-fronted flats, all facing south (sort of greenhouses – known as sun-spaces) to absorb the heat, keeping everyone warm – even in the winter. The second floor is made of carved, curved wood, bulging out of the glass porch, giving the impression of tree houses. At the very top, on the roof, are lush, riotous gardens. The rows of buildings have a cobblestoned space (not for cars) between them so kids can play safely because everyone can see them. Even if you don't care about the zero carbon emissions, there are other benefits: the residents care about each other. You need help? The whole place has your back. You want privacy, you have your own piece of land to grow what your heart desires, and if you want to mingle, there are communal dinners and social nights where the inmates dance to live music. Everyone looked happy. Maybe they put it on for me and, when I left, they all became bitches again, but I doubt it.

So, there you have it, green shoots growing in London, which shows that if you create the infrastructure people will come and once they have tried a place like this – built on good intentions – they will get a taste for this kind of life.

Intentional Communities/Ecovillages

If living in a city isn't for you, rural ecovillages are now becoming the last word in communal living. These already exist so you don't have to hunt in a haystack. I have the Communities Directory, it's about four inches thick filled with thousands of intentional communities and co-housing projects in almost every country in the world. The plan is to build 77,000 new ecohomes by 2024. I visited a few communities and even though there are problems, they deliver what it says on the tin. I'm not a natural-born eco-person – I fly, I drive, I do other bad, non-greeny things – but I'm sick to death of listening to conversations at dinner parties about what a shame it is that the world is going to melt in ten years. Now that I'm 'woke' I've started to say to these verbal do-gooders, 'Get off the pot or shut up. If you're so upset by the world, go off-grid and Thoreau-it-up.'

These intentional communities shouldn't be confused with the communes of the 1960s where it was all about free sex and sharing pans of beans. Even though that's where they started. I wanted to live in a commune back then but alas was too young and my parents would have killed me. There was one called 'The Pig Farm' which had an entrance lined with ten Cadillacs buried in the sand; the front parts deep in the ground, the tails jutting straight up into the air. Why they did this, I have no idea. I guess if you're stoned enough it makes sense. Anyway, it's probably good that I was too young, I'd be a casualty from bad acid by now.

Nowadays, the old-fashioned commune where an orgy was just another night in has been replaced by a group of like-minded people who want to create a carbon-free, zero-emissions, sustainable community. The villages are well designed; sleek, gorgeously landscaped wooden houses surrounded by lush flower and vegetable gardens. Unlike in the past, the residents don't just sit around on cat-hair sofas smoking weed, they work in nearby towns or from home. I'm sure they still smoke weed but they have jobs and a fully functioning brain.

To get to the roots of the intentional community move-ment we have to find the Mother of all of them . . . and she is in Scotland, near Inverness.

Findhorn Community

It was founded in 1962, doing eco before it was even a word. I won't go into too much detail as to how the place started because you might just shut this book, never to open it again, or think I've gone off with the fairies (literally, because they played a big part in the beginning). So trust me on this and keep reading because fifty-seven years later, what started as a pioneering intentional community in the early 1960s has turned into a hotbed of serious innovation that just might be able to save us and the planet.

History of Findhorn

It was love at first sight when Eileen clapped eyes on the very dapper, blue-eyed Flight Lieutenant Peter Caddy of the RAF (they would become the founders of Findhorn). She was a mumsy housewife sewing on buttons, married to another RAF officer. She didn't leave her husband simply because she fancied the blue-eyed one, it was because they found that they both shared a vision and they were highly spiritual and believed they had a joint higher purpose. (Okay, this is where I get off the bus.) It turns out, as it happens, that Eileen had a direct hotline to God so she received messages from Him and passed them straight on to Peter who then planned what they would do next. (I'm immediately imagining saying to my husband, 'Go wash the dishes, God told me to tell you.' And him telling me to 'Fuck off.')

Peter and Eileen were offered a job in the north of

Scotland, managing a hotel, Cluny House, a one-hundred-bedroomed place that needed more than a little work done on it. They were very successful for a while but eventually Peter was fired because he was making his decisions based on Eileen's messages from God and in the hospitality biz that just doesn't cut it.

With nowhere else to go, they moved into a nearby caravan park, living in a two-room trailer about fifteen by eight feet, and sharing it with their three children (did I mention she had children with Peter?) and their friend, Dorothy. Even more challenging, they were parked in some sand dunes, usually in gale-force-ten winds, next to a garbage dump. Eileen at this point couldn't hear what God was trying to say, what with all the noise in the caravan and the wind bashing the tin walls, so God suggested she go to the municipal toilet block between four and six in the morning. Of course, Eileen obeyed and sat on the loo at those hours picking up messages from above. She was told something like, 'Build a magic garden and the people will come and this will become a great community, a city of light.' All this from the loo.

Eileen's message was to let Dorothy guide them on the garden, where and what to plant. Dorothy had no previous experience in horticulture; however, she could now also pick up gardening advice from plant spirits called 'devas' and, to everyone's astonishment, vegetables sprung from the sand; not just normal ones, but cabbages weighing in at forty-two pounds. Soil experts visited, shook their heads saying it was impossible, and declared it a miracle, and so the people began to come . . . in droves. Like the vegetable version of Woodstock, it attracted hundreds of, probably stoned, New Agers.

You would imagine Eileen looked like Janis Joplin, with nervous-wreck hair, wild eyes and a vodka bottle sewn on to her lips, but no, with a prim pair of spectacles and a perm, Eileen might have been mistaken for anyone's grandmother. Every night she and Peter changed for dinner and insisted all residents do likewise. (Let's picture this: Peter in a kilt, Eileen in an evening gown and the other guests in never-washed-before kaftans and bird feathers.) By the late 1970s, mixed among the 'unkempt crowd', as Eileen called them, were people who shared her vision, guided by the direction of the 'clear small voice within'. Over the years, it slowly crept from what was referred to as 'The Vatican of the New Age' to what it is now: the global centre of ecological innovation and sustainability.

No longer a simple caravan park, the community now has 600 residents and 1–2,000 extras living outside in the old Cluny hotel and the village of Findhorn but still part of the foundation.

The houses come in all shapes and sizes, made of shingled, multicoloured wood, heated by solar panelling and biomass heaters (woodchip-fuelled boilers); waste is turned into clean water and all rubbish is boiled and recycled into a fertilized soil where flowers now bloom. This means your shit can eventually grow a garden.

Findhorn is set in woodland (remember, all grown on sand), with actual neighbourhoods; some swanky, some affordable housing, many made with turf growing on the roofs, some made of wooden whisky barrels. There are meditation areas, schools, offices, organic gardens, a 600-seat theatre, cafes, art studios; clearly God knows a thing or two about landscaping and architecture. A higgledy-piggledy path connects them all, a little like in the land of Oz. The population is made up of paid workers, lawyers, business people, therapists, doctors, entrepreneurs, artists, the elderly, babies and everyone in between.

Day 1

My friend and editor, Joanna Bowen, went to Findhorn with me. I was writing about it so we were given the place of honour to stay in, Eileen's final resting place. One of her children lovingly built her a beautiful two-bedroom house crafted to perfection. It was in this house that we found books about her life and, let me be honest, I was completely spooked. I was sleeping in her bed and got paranoid that she didn't like me being there. I assumed even though she was dead, she'd know I was a non-believer and would return to kill me. First, she clearly tried to freeze me to death because there was no heating. They told me it was turned on, but these people are so hearty, some of them wear shorts (it was zero degrees in December) so they don't feel the elements like a Princess does. They brought me heaters and I turned the place into a sauna, which I know Eileen was furious about. Isn't that strange, I don't believe she talked to God and there I was talking to her. So I went to sleep that first night, terrified.

Day 2

Each morning there's optional group meditation so I'm sitting there for half an hour, not calm at all but frozen like a solid block of fear. I detected a flicker of breath so I knew I was alive, otherwise, frozen. My teeth were actually chattering and in this state I went back to Eileen's. Janet, our guide, said that many people from London are shaken up the first day from suddenly dropping into this strange new land where everything moves at half-speed and everyone's nice, so you feel safe. Now you can start to feel things other than that slowly percolating anxiety. And what I felt was pure panic. After a while, having cooled down emotionally, I thought back on my normal routines and I came to the conclusion that I'm insane.

48 Hours Earlier: An Example of My Life

Two days ago, I did a mindfulness talk for MI5 in the morning (it seems they're under a little stress) and in the afternoon I spoke to 500 tube builders in their bright-orange vests and hard hats who were digging the new underground station at Vauxhall and Battersea. It seems they're under a little stress too, so much so that there are more suicides in this job than any other. (They work outrageous hours and literally don't see daylight because their shifts are so long.) I asked if they felt it difficult to tell someone when they felt they might be approaching the edge? They were silent. I guess they don't talk about their feelings much in a black hole halfway under London. Then one of the more hulky men stood up and proudly announced, 'I have my friends here, there they are [he pointed at them]. I told them I wanted to kill myself. I even went to the bridge and planned how I would jump. I talked about it to my friends and they talked me out of it. I know they really care about me and I care about them.' May I say the whole room burst into applause. At the end, I suggested we do a little mindfulness and I thought they would surely protest . . . but no, I looked up and I could see 500 hard-hatted hard guys with eyes shut, calmly breathing.

I had to run from that to get a train to somewhere in Wales to do a show that night. I missed my stop because

I was writing this book, didn't understand the Welsh station announcement (I thought someone was coughing up a hairball) and realized I wasn't going to make it to the theatre on time. A woman on the train heard me panicking/yelping over the phone to my stage manager, phoned her husband, who met me at the next station, and they drove me at top speed to the theatre. Such is humanity on a good day. I gave them tickets to the show and kissed their feet many times.

Then yesterday I took a train back to London from the north to change trains to get to another show I was doing in the south. Anyway, when I got on that train, I realized with a zapper to the heart that my computer was missing. I bounded off and barked at some railroad person to point me to the lost-and-found. So, holding multiple overloaded bags, I hunch-backed-of-Notre-Dame raced there to find the lost-and-found, which can't even find itself, it's so hidden – it's easier to locate Narnia. Both of my lungs collapsed on the run back and I heard my back cracking under the weight. I made it to the show and afterwards we went to a dress-up party in an art gallery, staying over at a friend of a friend's house before leaving for Findhorn.

So I suppose Janet may have had a point that my body was informing me it wanted a divorce.

Day 3

In the afternoon, I went to join a mindfulness session with a group of locals with learning disabilities. They come to Findhorn once a week, do gardening and then meditation. We all walked over from the dining room with the kids with Tourette's shouting and others making noises, then we went into the meditation room and when the gong gonged, there wasn't a peep. Total silence as they sat focused on their breathing. After the gong to mark the session was over, the noise began again. I almost cried. It was so profound.

How inspiring to discover that Findhorn has evolved from the old giant-cabbage-miracle days to a community with the highest concentration of social enterprises in the UK (over forty-five). One of those projects is GEN – a UN-recognized enterprise creating environmentally sustainable communities around the world. Some of the founders have become world leaders in creating a vision for future living; I have chosen GEN as one of my world savers in the last chapter of this book.

Though I can't completely buy into the conversations Eileen Caddy had with God fifty years ago, she was certainly inspired when she said, 'If you want to do something to help the world situation, look within. As you change your consciousness to love, peace, harmony and unity, the consciousness of the whole world will change.'

I ended up loving Findhorn and if it wasn't plonked so far up north, with those freezing-your-nose-off winter conditions, I would seriously think about moving there for the same reason other people go: to find a new way of living where we all feel included instead of isolated in our cold and lonely silos of self-absorption.

Anglian Water

Big business is also now getting involved in building communities. I saw it in action when Joanna and I went to see a project set up by Anglian Water to resurrect a failing community. They chose the town of Wisbech by looking on the map of the 'Indices of Deprivation' (I had no idea it existed), which is like the *X Factor* for the worst town in their area, and Wisbech won. Of a population of 30,000, 48 per cent are on a living wage working in potato-chip making, pea-canning or chicken-killing factories and, for academic achievement, they come in the bottom 10 per cent in the UK. The town is filled with immigrants from Eastern Europe, many of whom have seasonal picking work. There was no railway station, no cinema and hardly any shops. I was told that many of the girls' ambition is to get pregnant. The boys leave school early because there are no jobs, so there is no point. All together, it was a demoralized place.

Anglian Water have started to turn the place around, working with key residents to help create a thriving community centre, organizing a training programme which leads to apprenticeships and jobs, and setting up a homeless shelter. The community has changed and is starting to thrive, and it was astounding to see what big business can do for the good.

And that, folks, is what the next chapter is all about.

2

Business

I've never understood business. What do business people do besides take meetings and try to sell something? There's that corporate-speak jargon I've been told they use at strategic-trans-sector, peer-to-peer, co-creating, brainstorm meetings, meaning nothing to me and probably most of the people who use it – you've heard them talking, saying stuff like: 'Open the kimono', 'Drink the Kool-Aid', 'Re-evaluate the matrix'. Here's a funny one: 'corporate values' – what would a value be besides making as much as you can, as fast as you can? I am sometimes asked to give out prizes at company award ceremonies where the HR team all whoop as one of their colleagues weeps and wobbles her way to the stage to accept the trophy (a shard of Perspex) for the 'best sanitation department in Woolcock'. So for me to be writing about business is, at least, amusing.

Where We Are Now

Let's all agree that the world of business doesn't rap at this moment in time. We are no longer impressed by the success of the rich as it is shoved in our faces; it now inflames our sense of injustice. Here are some of the facts that should empty your bowels:

- 1 per cent of the world have the same amount of money as 99 per cent of the world put together.
- Forty-two people hold the same wealth as 3.7 billion of the world's poorest.
- The entire wealth of Jeff Bezos, owner of Amazon (my home-away-from-home for binge shopping at 4 a.m. for things I will never need), has increased to $122 billion. Just to give you an idea of how much that is, the whole of government spending in Ethiopia with a population of 105 million people is a mere $95 billion. Why Ethiopians aren't hunting him down, I do not know.
- In 1978 the average CEO made about thirty times more than the average worker's salary. By 2006 the CEOs have seen almost a 950 per cent increase in their earnings. Meanwhile, the average American worker has seen an 11 per cent raise.

Bad News About Business

Okay, sorry, here's a little bad news just so you know where we are now: our work is killing us faster than wars, murderers and terrorists.

- An excess of 120,000 deaths in the UK have a work-related cause.
- Over £100 billion is lost each year in employee absenteeism due to stress.
- There are two words which have had to be created in Japanese and Chinese (*karoshi* and *guolaosi*) to describe 'death by work'. In Japan, around 10,000 people die from work-related causes every year. (I swear I'm not going to keep giving you more depressing news.)

My Story

My father was the quintessential, first-generation American businessman; he knew how to sell high, through charm and razor-sharp savvy, and buy low by ripping you off while you were sleeping. I assumed this was just business as normal: ruthless, cut-throat and may the biggest shyster in the trough win. I'd listen in on my dad as he pimped his sheep bladders. (That's what sausage casings are made of and that's what he unashamedly sold.) I once heard him say (he never conquered Americanisms), 'Well, dat's the vey the chicken crumbles.' Pretending to be light-hearted and jokey with a customer, I heard him say, 'Hey, Barbara, how many abortions have you had this week?' It seemed to work (maybe the buyers were as crass as he was). My father was known as the Casing King of the animal bladder and intestine world. (I was so mortified, I told everyone he was a fashion designer for hot dogs, it sounded less coarse.)

So, I was raised in the belief that the most conniving wins. My dad was a killer who took no prisoners in either his private or business life. If you ever ripped him off or tried to take advantage, he would hunt you down and make you squeal like a pig. He lovingly passed his wisdom on to me, telling me to screw people before they screwed me, so I just assumed this was how humans roll. If you ripped him off, he would leave the kind of greeting card someone did when they put a horse's head in bed with the guy who did the mob wrong in *The Godfather*.

It's ironic that both democracy and capitalism were actually designed to generate the highest possible opportunity for all. And it's true that when the capitalist system is motivated by generosity and kindness, the result is inclusiveness and creativity. However, when it's motivated by fear and greed, the result is the oppression of minorities, the condemnation of immigrants, greed, exploitation and a big, wide chasm between winners and losers.

Over the last twenty-five years, the gap between rich and poor has widened and the effect of this inequality isn't just the cranking up of the have-nots' envy, it's also affecting the haves. Once they make their pile they become obsessed with keeping it and building on it and so they hunker down into their egotistical 'it's all about me' state. These narcissists are the very people who cause the most harm in the world; fighting imagined enemies, kicking the underdog and believing that while their view is reality, the rest of us are deluded. These Hulk-like powermongers don't waste any energy caring about others and so are now the masters of global enterprises and presidents of nations. You can usually spot them: they're not only humourless but humanless and they don't mind being hated, they feed on it.

I'm not knocking making money, far from it. (I'm not writing this book for nothing.) The free market of capitalism has made it possible to live longer, be better educated, live healthier, with more medical breakthroughs, less starvation, etc. . . . so what's the problem? With all these goodies, life should be a bowl of cherries. So what's with all the loneliness, opioid addiction, alcoholism, depression, suicide and a dying planet?

The reason I'm discussing business is because it's becoming far more powerful than most political systems. While most government piggy banks are empty, business is rolling in it. Corporations run the politicians, who obey their beck and call. If an oil company wants more oil, the government will declare a war to get more. The enemy is only the enemy because they're sitting on the gold that you want. While I'm on the topic of gold, I thought you might like to know where we even got the idea of money in the first place. Even if you don't, I'll tell you anyway.

A Little Interlude – The History of Money

In days of way back, in olde yore times, we could use anything to pay for stuff: bullocks for big purchases and for the equivalent of small change, there were guinea pigs. People found these animals were too heavy to carry about so coins made of gold and silver replaced them.

Coins were being used all the way back in 2000 BC in the Middle East. We know this from ancient stories, like that a man was fined half a kilo of silver for biting off someone's nose (I did not make this up). A few hundred centuries later the Romans had the idea of minting coins and their first minting press in Rome was by the Temple of Juno Moneta – hence the word 'money'.

No one wanted to travel with gold or silver coins for fear of being mugged so you gave your money to a man in the market who would keep it safe for a small fee. (Why no one mugged these guys I do not know.) The moneymen did their business from benches in the marketplace and these were known as banks (bench in Latin is *bancus*). If one of these bankers robbed you (and when didn't they?), you would smash and rupture their bank (bench) – hence the word 'bankrupt'.

Enter the Jews

In medieval times, Christian theology proclaimed that charging interest was sinful, so very few went into the finance biz. Guess who stepped in? You guessed it – the Jews.

For centuries, Jews ran the money market for the European aristocracy's projects. In the 1760s, the savviest one, Mayer Amschel Rothschild, made a killing. Jews have not made a great name for themselves throughout history, except for the name Rothschild. To this day, everyone wants to be a Rothschild or marry one. The rest of the money-lending Jews were not as lucky with their stereotyping (see Shylock in *The Merchant of Venice*).

Next came the Industrial Revolution where all the rage was capitalism and the world changed for evermore. In the US you had the creation of railroads, steam engines and fleets of ships run by the industrial giants – Vanderbilt, Carnegie and Rockefeller (known as 'robber barons' back then; it does what it says on the tin) – who exploited the teeming poor as cheap labour to build their empires. They also built hospitals, universities and libraries, but in my opinion it was to appease their guilt so they wouldn't go to hell for exploiting the have-nots all in the name of free enterprise (free for whom, do you think?).

In 1891, Pope Leo summed up what was going on: 'Hence, by degrees it has come to pass that working men have been surrendered, isolated and helpless, to the hardheartedness of employers and the greed of unchecked competition.'

Twentieth Century

Obviously after two world wars there were limited resources and when that happens guess who doesn't get dinner? You guessed it. The workers. In some places they revolted and everywhere socialism grew in popularity; in the twentieth century, unions were created to protect the workers' rights. So capitalism was reined in for a moment . . . but that lasted ten minutes because business couldn't do business as usual what with the strikes and the continuous moaning of workers about their measly pay and appalling work conditions. Enter Reagan and Thatcher, who put their capitalist feet down and said a unified 'Fuck off' to the workers.

Okay, it really got down and dirty here when Milton Friedman, Nobel Prize-winning economist and father of what's known as modern capitalism, declared in 1970: 'The social responsibility of business is to increase its profit. Businessmen who take seriously their responsibilities for providing employment, eliminating discrimination, avoiding pollution . . . are preaching pure and unadulterated socialism.' It wasn't until 'Milton the mad' came along that capitalism took a new path. He advocated that bosses charge the highest price for their products while paying their workers the least to make a maximum killing. The *Oxford Dictionary* definition of capitalism (and what Milton shouts from the rooftops) is: 'An economic and political system in which a country's trade and industry are controlled by private owners for profit.' Eventually, what became law was that those who invest in the company (the shareholders) could legally demand more profit each year or else they could sue the company. The law would protect the shareholder in case the company went bankrupt or was involved in fraud. The CEO's job was to do whatever it took to raise the stock prices no matter what the consequences were on stakeholders (employees and customers, society and the environment).

The 1980s was the time of Neoliberalism when everything was about 'money, money, money', as Abba knew. Banks began to become big businesses, lending money at a fixed rate of interest (they stole this idea from the Jews). The word 'credit' comes from the word for belief so you had to believe that the bank would give you back your money when you asked for it and the bankers had to believe that you would pay the interest. Everyone crossed their fingers and said, like in *Peter Pan*, 'I do believe in fairies' to make Tinker Bell come back from the dead. Sometimes it worked, sometimes it didn't. Like when you'd show up but the bank had loaned your money to someone else, so you got nothing. It was as if, even with all your wishing, Tinker Bell had died. As soon as we stopped believing in banks and fairies, there was a big bad crash.

This is why we had heroes like Gordon Gekko, who proudly says in the film *Wall Street*, 'Greed is good . . . it's right . . . it works . . . It cuts through and captures the essence of the evolutionary spirit.' And everyone just loved Gordon. (The present President of the United States won because he's the brute of all brutes; he's Gekko, squared. If people think he is the fittest, we're fucked.)

Hubris finally brought us down in 1987 when we could suck no more out of an ignorant public, which led to the downfall of companies like General Motors, Sears and Enron, to name a few. But it was a skirmish compared with the 2008 financial disaster. Lehman Brothers, Citigroup, Fannie Mae and others who had been swindling the shareholders by 'over-leveraging' (announcing, due to an arrogance and narcissism the size of Texas, that they were loaded with money when in fact they had emptied the piggy bank with their failed short-term gambles) finally crashed and burnt.

Richard Fuld, CEO of Lehman Brothers, known as 'The

Gorilla', charmingly said, 'If anyone gets in my way, what I really want to do is reach in and rip out their heart and eat it before they die.' It's chilling that, unlike the fictitious character of Gekko, Richard Fuld actually exists in real life.

Status

In the name of status, as in working for a hot-shit brand, people are willing to work day, night and weekends to be able to say casually, 'Yeah, I work for Google.' Even if they're cleaning the toilets. They may try to dazzle you by saying they're the CEO of sanitation but really they're toilet cleaners. Status and money mean everything here in the twenty-first century, though they both can seriously damage your health.

Ask people if status or money makes them happy and chances are they'll shrug their shoulders and look a little sad about not having a home or social life, as if that's the inevitable result of the natural state of the world. But they would never complain about having no life, for fear that if they don't answer the call at four in the morning they'll be replaced by someone who will. I know so many people who admit they're unhappy and complain they have no 'me' time. Well, guess what? In the future you'll have all the 'me' time you want. And before you blow your top panicking about how you'll make a living, I have a suggestion. What if jobs that we think are menial now, such as caring for the old, sick or ill, were rewarded with a nice salary so that these roles became as cool as wearing £700 sneakers or driving a Porsche? Working in the service of others could become a status symbol that carries high prestige like being a head of a sexy start-up or a celebrity. There could be a kind of *Love Island* where people compete for who's done the kindest thing for another human being. As we are addicted to ranking, we could have a version of the Forbes rich list for those of us who give the most.

Some of the jobs that net the highest salaries don't add much value to our lives. Teachers (except in Finland), nurses and care workers make hardly anything and we need them more than corporate consultants (whatever the fuck they do). New York got it right with paying garbage collectors; they can take home $70,000 a year plus overtime and perks because they're the ones who keep the city running and everyone really needs them. On the other hand, if the corporate consultant stopped working no one would notice or care.

Why Did We Get So Greedy?

Sixty years ago, economist Victor Lebow said:

> Our enormously productive economy demands that we make consumption our way of life. That we convert the buying and use of goods into rituals, that we seek our spiritual satisfactions and our ego satisfactions, in consumption. We need things consumed, burnt up, worn out, replaced, and discarded at an ever-increasing pace.

Relentless consumption is needed, so the argument goes, just to maintain economic stability. Our identity becomes 'I am what I've got'.

For the last 150 years, we've been able to justify our greed by bringing out that old Darwinian catchphrase 'survival of the fittest'. This is the one that people trot out to justify their savage hunger for money and power.

In fact, the phrase only appeared in the fifth edition of *On the Origin of Species* to mean, 'better designed to fit with the local environment'. What Darwin actually meant by it was that those who cooperate best, survive longest. Teamwork is the winning strategy, not competition. So the fittest are the ones who bring people together and are the best liked.

Are We Really Natural Warmongers?

Another misconception we've all bought into is that war and aggression are also in our human DNA. Even Winston Churchill pumped up the idea: 'The story of the human race is War. Except for brief and precarious interludes, there has never been peace in the world: even before history began murderous strife was universal and unending.' We cling to this myth that humanity will be waging war forever and always has done.

Hundreds of thousands of years ago, we took care of everyone in our tribe; I mean everyone – the old, infirm, stupid, uninteresting and overweight. There was peace on earth because there was enough space to not bump into anyone else and plenty to eat; the land was our buffet and we could help ourselves (no having to fight for a buffalo wing). There was enough to feed the entire population of about 238.

It was when land and food got scarce that we began to declare war on each other because once we accumulated wealth we got a taste for all the stuff we could buy with it and we'd attack other groups for more. Ever since, what has motivated war, more than a blood-thirsty taste for killing, has been the desire for what the other tribe has.

Animals

Darwin assumed that if two closely related species showed the same behaviours under the same circumstances, the psychology behind it was similar so, under the skin, animals and humans are in sync. When a chimp is injured other chimps will help to calm him or her down by kissing or grooming them. And once a chimp makes a friend, once it picks a single nit off another ape, they are locked into an everlasting friendship. Of course, we don't lick or pick nits off each other but we, like them, have the proclivity to care. (I have eaten nits occasionally and they are delicious.) When competitors do fight for status or power, they often just posture by beating their chests (just like rugby players doing the hakahukka) and avoid bloodshed, unless it's a life-or-death scenario.

You want to see animals with feelings? Go watch Attenborough's last series, *Dynasties*, where a lioness goes back into enemy territory to lick the wounds of a lion who was injured in battle when trying to defend her. You'll weep like a baby when you see elephants mourn their dead and sometimes carry the bones of the deceased for months, unable to part with them.

They chose the wrong animal when they came up with the *Wolf of Wall Street*, because wolves live in packs and care for their young and the sick. They fight over territory and food but really it's for the sake of the pack. A violent nature doesn't mean they don't have the possibility of having empathy. It turns out that it's not a dog-eat-dog world, even if you're a dog.

It was primatologist Jane Goodall who said that you have to live with animals in nature to see what actually happens. After years of close observation, she discovered, contrary to popular perception, that female apes aren't turned on by the alphas. Turns out they sneak to the edge of their tribe's territory and secretly mate with a beta. They're not aware of the reason but nature favours genetic diversity . . . and nature rules. If everyone mated with the alpha, everyone in the tribe would be cousins and all would have anger issues. Meanwhile, the alpha, thinking it's his baby, protects it with his life. I don't know the ape word for 'sucker' but that's what he is.

So as I said, Darwin found that animals are basically highly cooperative, believe in fairness and are mostly peace loving. And if animals hunt in packs and share the goods, why shouldn't it be natural for us to do that too?

Even though the title of Richard Dawkins's book *The Selfish Gene* seems to indicate that genes are selfish, he didn't mean they spend their days hunting each other down. Genes are described by scientists today as 'social in nature': 'Organisms get information from the environment and from each other on how to change. The conditions, the culture and connectivity are as important as the actual code.'

By the way, the person who coined 'survival of the fittest' was Herbert Spencer, a nineteenth-century philosopher. He and the following generations of libertarians (Hayek, Friedman, Thatcher) used it to justify their views on 'society' being meaningless and that all freedom should be granted to individuals to do whatever came naturally to them; fairness and social ethics were out the window. The slogan was adopted by him to convince people that human beings are naturally warlike and that we were built to compete and fight. It was poverty that stopped progress and, inevitably, if you have a winner, there has to be a loser. It was convenient for the powerful to believe this myth because they didn't have to feel responsible for something that they convinced themselves was just a biological fact.

Most people who are powerful and unimaginably wealthy have been trained to react and think like a reptile even though they are delightful to meet and probably generous and kind to their friends. Most City bankers admit they're overpaid and that teachers and nurses are underpaid but they are institutionalized and can no longer imagine a life outside their bubble.

And speaking of bubbles, in the 1980s around the time the bubble burst, I remember meeting someone working at a hedge fund who told me that every month there would be a performance review and if they weren't pulling their weight (meaning that for whatever reason they were in the bottom 10 per cent), they would be told to clear their desk and take a hike. During the crash, the streets were littered with the newly fired, bemused and bewildered like zombies banging into each other, carrying their desks in boxes. Those who kept their jobs began to work ungodly hours and weekends, never off the phone, terrified their heads were the next to roll, so they became even more cut-throat. This was the time, through the 1990s, when salaries of bosses went off the scale and, to add a little cream, they were getting huge bonuses. In order to keep their corporate structure working they needed a workforce which was frightened of being ousted and therefore uncomplaining and at the same time was being motivated to join in the party by having the carrot of success dangled in front of them. 'You too can have what I have' was the subliminal message, 'as long as you work like a dog and suck up all the shit I'm throwing at you.' It was a culture of cruelty that was prevalent in a lot of financial institutions at the time and even though there are remaining vestiges of this corporate culture, I am happy to notice that we are moving away from that paradigm.

So Here Come the Green Shoots

Muhammad Yunus, the Nobel Prize-winning economist, stated that, 'Indifference to other human beings is deeply embedded in the framework of economics but a true human being can be selfless, caring, sharing and community-building.' He goes on to ask the question I will answer in this chapter, 'How do we create companies that help to promote our good sides?' Hard to believe but it appears that caring about the employees has lately become the house style of a few evolved corporations, making the workers feel they matter and that their welfare is crucial to their companies; these are now being referred to as 'healing organizations'. I like what Ian McCallum, a South African physician and naturalist, says: 'We have to stop speaking about the Earth being in need of healing. The Earth doesn't need healing, we do.'

This care for each other at work is a far step from the old 'control and command' model which focused only on hitting performance targets. The cynical side of me thinks, 'Yeah, they're keeping their employees sweet so they can drive them even harder and longer.' It appears I'm wrong, which is so rare for me. Frederic Laloux ranked different styles of corporate behaviour in his book *Reinventing Organizations*, from greedy self-interest to caring collaboration.

1. The greed-based version of capitalism states, 'Here's an opportunity to make money regardless of whether it involves exploiting a need or gap in the marketplace and regardless of the human consequence.' PS This is the model that has been prevalent in banking for about forty years.

2. A slightly more evolved mindset says, 'Here is an opportunity to make money by exploiting a need or gap in the market but we will initiate some corporate social-responsibility initiatives and employee wellness programmes to help the struggling.'

3. A better system in business would say, 'Here's an opportunity to make a profit while serving the stakeholders' (customers, communities, workers) needs.'

4. A healing organization says, 'In a quest to alleviate suffering and elevate joy, we serve the needs of all stakeholders; our employees, customers, communities and environment. We seek to continually improve the lives of stakeholders while making a profit so we can continue to grow and heal.'

I don't know whether this last model exists outside of Paradise but maybe I'll find an example.

Why is Change Suddenly Happening?

The millennials are the first generation to grow up with social media so they can communicate globally faster than the speed of sound and create a new meme in moments, in contrast to older generations who took two hundred years going from plough to automobile. They could have dumped the ox in a few hours because they can adapt and reinvent so quickly.

So having had it with the boomer generation, whose credo is of the 'rape and loot' school of business, they've come up with their own blueprint almost overnight.

Millennials or Generation Y believe sharing and contributing to the common good is the way to go to have a good life. TrendWatching.com said of them and the following Generation Z: 'They are accelerating a cultural shift where "giving is already the new taking".' Here are the statistics:

- 61 per cent of 13–30-year-olds feel personally responsible for making a difference in the world

- 83 per cent will trust a company more if it's socially and environmentally responsible
- Volunteering by college students increased by 20 per cent between 2002–2005
- 83 per cent volunteered to help in some way in 2005

Nowadays it's starting to seem as if it's all about the fittest being the kindest.

My own generation began with the belief in equality and fairness but now, as grown-ups, we've done exactly the same as the 'establishment' were doing back then . . . you know, the one which we were rebelling against. In other words, since the 1960s, we, the Boomers, have looted the planet blind, using the earth as an ashtray; it's not surprising our kids are disgusted by what we've done.

I know some big businesses are trying to patch things up by 'going green'. Maybe installing a wind machine in the men's loo to replace a hand dryer or telling the employees that if they don't flush the toilet, they'll get a bonus at Christmas. Now we have carbon 'offsets' like, when you fly, you promise to plant a few trees. There's probably a desk at the airport where they give you a packet of seed on arrival. This is known as 'greenwashing' and while it is a nod to a shared responsibility for the planet, it really just soothes the corporate guilty pang, like sucking an antacid.

Decades ago, most people got work once they left school, stayed with a company for life or nearly life and when they left they were handed a retirement cheque and a gold watch. Oh, by the way, they didn't burn out because they worked from 9 a.m to 6 p.m., had weekends (phone free because there were no mobiles) and had holidays three times a year. (Those were the good old days.) You can see why the younger generation are quaking in their pants. After the 1980s' debacle they felt frightened that whatever job they got was precarious. Jobs in the old sense have become scarce since then. Even if you go to university, you will struggle to find that kind of job for life. I read in the papers that a third of 20–34-year-olds, mostly men, still live in their childhood bedrooms. So, for some reason the millennials don't seem to approve of what the older generations have done to the earth. It upsets them that nitrogen and phosphorus from fertilizer is in our water supply, carbon dioxide is at its highest level in 600,000 years and still increasing, causing floods, devastating storms, extreme temperatures, the drying-up of rivers, deforestation, acidified oceans, pollution and the culling of species at a rate of 200 a day. What's their problem? Millennials are aware of these facts while most of the old dinosaurs choose to turn their fat cheeks the other way, thinking, 'I'm going to be dead by the time the shit hits the fan so why stop shopping?'

My Story

During my student days, I partook in many a riot, trying to shut down the big corporations who supported the Vietnam War or were polluting the air or just being greedmongers. We wanted everyone in the world to be equal and for everyone to get a fair share. We were eco before eco became chic, saving the planet before we trashed it. Many lived in communes, growing their own vegetables and making the smallest ever footprint because no one worked and they were all sharing a stained mattress smoking organic pot. At university, I shouted with the best of them, 'Ho Ho Ho Chi Minh,' waving a red book. I wasn't sure what was in it but it looked good with my outfit (Chinese military). My

> whole generation spent its youth fighting the anti-establishment cause. And now look what's happened? We are the establishment.

Conscious Capitalism

Having been burnt by us elders, the millennials have seen what unleashed greed leads to and have learnt the lesson of what not to do, so they're motivated by mission and purpose rather than money. It's all about saving the planet, giving aid to people in dire need and working to live rather than living to work.

While researching this book I've seen in the flesh with my own eyes what's happening in business and I know a phoenix is rising out of the ashes of the dying old economic model and being born as a whole new paradigm called 'conscious capitalism'. Remember, I'm talking about tiny green shoots so don't give me, 'Well, it's not happening at HSBC. They still need to make profits.' I'm not an idiot and nor are they, people need to pay taxes on profits otherwise the economy skids to a halt.

But work should also give people something that would improve their lives and it's not just money. This new model of business is number 4 (see above) from the book *Reinventing Organizations*, where it reads, 'Caring for the well-being of the employees, customers and everyone on the supply chain, helping the local community and protecting nature.' Employees want 'purpose' now, not just profit, and this new sensibility began because of a widespread awareness of the environmental crisis. The idea that your children's children may not have a planet to walk on makes slaving your lifetime for money seem pointless. It's not brand new – over a century ago Bernard Shaw said:

This is the joy in life: being used for a purpose recognized by yourself as a mighty one, being a force of Nature instead of a feverish, selfish clod of ailments and grievances, complaining that the world will not devote itself to making you happy.

John Mackey, CEO of Whole Foods Market, and Raj Sisodia PhD coined the phrase and wrote the book *Conscious Capitalism*. In it they say that business should focus more on purpose than on pure profit, cooperation rather than competition. When I say conscious capitalism, don't picture some old hippy giving away pickles at the side of the road, what's new is that it's going mainstream; as far back as 2013, the *Harvard Business Review* showed that 'Companies that practice "conscious capitalism" perform ten times better than their peers.'

Younger people want to have a better work life than we did and since most of our lives are spent at work, why not use that time too to help us find meaning and even happiness? I hear people saying they'll find meaning when they have time, maybe on the weekend, on holiday or when they retire. But there is a growing sense that we have to find it right now, otherwise we're wasting our breathing time on earth. These conscious companies aim to do just that and some even focus on creating a feeling of happiness which, because emotions are infectious, can spread like a contagion. If the team has a mission to make the world better, it feels good (all acts of generosity do) and then that feeling ripples from person to person throughout the organization.

All the books about this reimagined capitalism talk about finding a meaningful purpose. I had no idea what purpose meant in a business context, I thought it was like the word 'value' that they bandy about – some more junk jargon. I looked it up: 'A compelling purpose reduces the friction within an organization because it gets everybody pointing in the same direction.' When everyone gets passionate about the same mission, they become part of a 'team human' community and that's when people start being driven by their hearts rather than their wallets.

So here we have the hierarchy of principles of a conscious-capitalist company:

1. **Purpose** refers to the difference you try to make in the world

2. **Mission** is the way in which you will achieve that purpose

3. **Vision** is the picture your company shares of what the world will look like once your purpose has been achieved

I would never have dreamt that these principles could be found in a list of what matters in the office. If I had known when I was in school that this change was coming, I would have cooled it on the rioting. I would have told everyone that someday capitalism (which was our sworn enemy) is going to change its feathers. They wouldn't have believed me though so I could have saved my breath.

Another Thing About Conscious Capitalism

In his book, Raj says:

> Think of a caterpillar transforming into a butterfly. In the early stages it just eats and nothing much changes except it grows one hundred times its original size. When the time is right, it enters a cocoon phase and then emerges as a

butterfly, not only beautiful but useful, it pollinates plants, producing food for others to live off, playing its part in Nature.

This can be applied to humans and corporations; we can just stay like grubbing caterpillars, consuming all we can with no price to pay. But we can also transform and create value for others while making the world more beautiful. Needless to say, I was confused by this metaphor, not knowing what it feels like to be a caterpillar, especially a conscious one. Raj goes on:

> Unlike caterpillars we can't wait for nature to trigger our evolution to a higher consciousness, we have to raise our own consciousness and make deliberate choices that make us more caring.

Where do you find a butterfly in business, I wanted to know? He pointed me to one and it is called Patagonia – not the region in South America, the sportswear clothing company. For a moment, I thought I'd have to fly to Argentina but it's in Ventura, California, still twelve hours away but I had to see it; it's the movie star who just won the Oscar of conscious capitalism.

Patagonia: A Star is Born

It's been called the coolest company on the planet. The story of it is in a book called *Let My People Go Surfing*. I said before, part of my mission in writing this book was to be inspired to change my life, maybe I would live in an ecovillage or teach kids in Finland, but now I thought, maybe I'll get a job at Patagonia. Also, it was winter in the UK while I was writing this part so it was doubly crucial I go to California.

Having arrived, I had to drive for two hours from LA to Ventura in a desert landscape, passing a series of oases full of nail bars and fast-food outlets, separated by continents of parking lots, but when I got out, there was the ocean, smooth, gold-tinged, sunsetting, surfer dudes riding the pipeline (like I know what that is). I was happy already. The next day I met Vincent Stanley, a co-founding employee who's been with the company since the beginning, more than forty-five years ago. Patagonia is not like the Google headquarters in the UK, all showy-offy. Google's interiors are eclectic with varying environments. Some decorator must be on Ayahuasca. One area is based on a Miami hotel lobby, that leads to a Brazilian jungle, then your grandmother's house (flowered wallpaper and rocking chairs), next a womb room where the chairs are big round balls, with a slot you enter to work in a padded birth sack. No one working there would notice any of this because their foreheads are glued to keyboards. Anyway, the Patagonia buildings are two-storeyed and made of old wood like a Southwestern ranch. Surrounding the buildings are natural landscapes (no fountains or manicured lawns, looking like they've just had a bikini wax like most business campuses I've seen). No tree has been cut down to make room for any building so some grow in the buildings. Between them are spaces where they have created playing areas and schools. They bring their kids into work, starting from babies age three months (I'm sure there's also a place where the womenfolk can birth their babies straight into a sandbox) up to age ten. Day care and school are subsidized for the employees' kids and you can hear them laughing and playing wherever you are. I was told the presence of kids makes adults more conscious of who they're changing the world for. I noticed surfboards leaning against some of the walls. I guess when someone shouts, 'Surf's Up!', people grab them and head for the beach to ride a windpipe (no idea).

And people here are very loyal. Out of the 300 at the Ventura premises, most are in their twenties to early forties, thirty people are over sixty and have been here over twenty years and five are still here from 1972.

I met Vincent in the cafeteria; wood walls and photos of people (probably the employees) in various dangerous sports positions: falling down a cliff in skis, riding the crest of a forty-foot wave, steering a sailboat through a tsunami. We sat at one of the many picnic tables where everyone mingles. People are dressed casually, looking happy and relaxed; the women are beautiful in a Joni Mitchell, flowing-long-hair kind of way. (No dye. Whoever sees anyone without dyed hair? Not me.) And get this. No make-up. The men are bronzed and blond, and here was Vincent looking like Sam Shepard (google him), the real, just-off-the-range, rugged-faced American cowboy, slow talkin' but razor mind, so I was in love. While he told me the story of Patagonia, I was trying not to dribble the alfalfa I was eating down my front.

I heard (entranced) how Yvon Chouinard (Vincent's uncle) fifty years ago was a climber scaling sheer vertical cliffs sometimes made of ice. He wasn't thinking about starting a clothing business. (Well, you wouldn't think of anything if dangling from a wall of ice.) At the time, he had no money so he and a friend lived in an abandoned incinerator, sometimes having to eat cat food, and was eventually jailed for having no place of residence. Incinerators didn't count. Anyway, in 1972 he went from selling climbing gear into clothing, mainly selling rugby shirts which were the only thing that wouldn't shred when scaling a peak. (Good to know because I'm always tearing my shirts when up Everest.) Eventually word went out about his mission to drop the wasteful and polluting model of doing business and 'build a new roof over the economy before the old decrepit one collapsed'.

So the people ('nonconformists and misfits') came from all over to work at Patagonia. Today they get 10,000 applicants for eighteen internships. Sixty per cent of vice presidents are women throughout the many outlets. Vincent said (and everything he says I agree with) that 'This generation has more in common with the hippy boomers than with any other generation.'

Here they walk the talk, believing they owe the earth a tax for the industrial impact of business, so each year since 1985 they have given away 10 per cent of all profits and since 2016 have given 100 per cent of Black Friday sales to local and global grassroot organizations, not big corporate charities. So far they've also given away $100 million since 1985 to about 2,500 grassroot environmental groups. When Trump said all businesses could have a tax cut, Patagonia gave theirs away, which was about $10 million.

And if you're running a big corporate organization and wondering how these guys make a profit, Patagonia's sales have quadrupled over the past decade. So rotate on that fact, Big Boys.

Patagonia is privately owned so they don't have to pay any return to the shareholder. Profits are shared with employees in a bonus pool. They work in groups where they can make independent decisions without always having to get approval from a higher being who might not know what's happening on the ground.

In their foreign-based supplier factories around the world – Vietnam, for example – auditors check to see if people are paid legally, work normal hours, have proper lighting, ventilation and medical aid.

Patagonia's other maxim is transparency not only to the

workers but to their competition. The theory goes that if everyone came clean about how they're doing business, they wouldn't be able to cut so many corners. For example, some companies would have to stop using Chinese children working by candlelight next to their arthritically damaged, overworked grandmothers because they'd have to report the conditions; there'll be blogs that will spread the word on who's abusing whom and, if your company is an offender, the customers will dry up. Fairly soon there will be an app (see chapter 4 on Technology) which you will use to check the provenance of the fabric, the carbon footprint and the amount of stress levels of the people who sewed it together. Transparency will be demanded by the public, it's the only way to build up trust. If companies come clean about their problems, everyone will be able to nip mistakes in the bud before they rot the tree. This was the case when, in the past, Patagonia found one of their products wasn't as harmless as they thought; they quickly admitted it and changed to a sustainable alternative and the result was that their fan base quadrupled.

Vincent walked me through the buildings, originally built in the 1980s with paintings of outdoor scenes on the walls. It's all cosy and piney and smells of Alpines, like an old-fashioned, homey ski resort. Everything seems organic and made of hemp. Ninety-five per cent of what was in that office is made of recycled materials, except me. He introduced me to very attractive, unstressed, smiling, white-teethed people, many working at waist-high desks where you stand to work. (This is why so many people have back pain because we [I] sit for a living and at some point in life can't get out of the chair.) I was nearly run over several times by giant dogs, I mean the size of horses, because no one has a Chihuahua like you'd see in Beverly Hills, they all have humongous canines running like the Pamplona bulls through the offices.

Vincent told me that people who grew up in 2000 or later want a higher mission and to use their intelligence and creativity for more than just the highest pay. No one wants to feel ashamed any more to name the company they work for. All the employees here are on the same mission: to help both the local community and global community . . . oh, and to make clothes. They all have an allocated time off to volunteer for things like saving salmon, irrigating land, breeding endangered species, cleaning rivers, teaching kids in third-world countries, saving whales, back-combing buffalos.

Yvon's decision to stick to his guns about keeping his company kosher was on the button. According to a recent survey of 40,000 shoppers in the US, 59 per cent are 'belief driven', meaning they want their money to make the world a better place. When they choose a brand they are starting to ask themselves if it's worth the social and environmental cost.

This could be because they've been made aware that if they don't stop the problem, they will have to swim to the malls through the flooding, burnt to a crisp from the now-menopausal climate while battling through hurricanes.

Vincent (my fiancé, in my mind) walked me to a 10,000-square-foot building containing the archives of Patagonia. Ellen and her assistant almost wept as they raved about the history, showing me photos of a topless Yvon in the 1960s forging those pitons or crampons (I thought they were related to sani-towels), you know, those steel spikes they use to pick their way up mountains. The other early employees looked like refugees from Woodstock, bell-bottoms and flowers in their hair.

They've had to become very conscientious about what products they use because the textile industry is one of the most chemically intensive industries on earth, second only to agriculture. Nearly 20 per cent of water pollution comes from dyeing and treatment. Some rivers in China, seen from the air, run indigo into the ocean because of the jeans I'm wearing.

They used to use conventionally grown cotton until they found out how harmful the chemicals are. (The cotton crop alone accounts for 10 per cent of the world's use of pesticides.) Organophosphates, linked to central nervous system damage in humans, is used as fertilizer, originally developed as nerve gas for the First World War. (So remember not to eat your hoodie.)

Each time Patagonia became aware of how much harm a garment made, they dumped it and started again. They switched entirely to organic cotton in 1996. But then they found that oil-based polyester could be made less harmful by using recycled sources rather than fresh oil so they made fleece jackets from twenty-five quart-sized plastic soda bottles melted down and extruded into fibre. (In the early days you got water from the tap straight into your mouth [some of you might remember] so you didn't have to worry about leftover plastic bottles.)

Now they're working on 'biomimicry regenerative practices'. (I have no idea what that means?) Maybe now sweaters are growing on trees and when you're done with them, you eat them. They also said (this isn't a joke) that they're converting abandoned fishing nets into sunglasses.

The main thing is not to waste, so Patagonia took out an ad in the *New York Times* that said, next to a picture of one of their jackets, 'Don't buy this jacket,' to discourage overconsumption. If something needs repairing, you send it back and it's repaired in one of the seventy-two repair centres, and if it really does reach the end, which is rare, they recycle

it and make something else out of it. If they can't repair it,
they send you a new one. I was told of one woman who
called in to say her fleece was peed on by a cat and could it be
replaced. The guy at the call centre said, 'Sure, what kind of
cat would you like?'

Needless to say, Vincent didn't propose but he gave me one
of my happiest days, where I realized that at least one company was doing what I dreamt about when I was eighteen. I
wanted a world where you could trust that people weren't
trying to screw you (I thank my father for instilling that one).
I still don't trust any government, but as I said before, business is what's going to change the world; politicians are too
busy running for office and then worrying about getting in
again or not being impeached (no names). So hurrah, Patagonia, for giving me faith, it's not the whole world yet but I'm
not looking for that, just a gold nugget in the mud, and you
are it. I love you, Vincent, if you're reading this.

B Corp

I think I've made it clear that customers, employees and
everyone down the supply chain to the little guy sewing in
Hanoi stay faithful to Patagonia because they trust it. So the
question is, are there other companies out there singing
from the same hymn sheet? Well, again thanks to the millennials and boomers with a conscience, the tide has turned
and now people want companies that benefit the world and
don't just suck out the resources, 'Wham bam, thank you,
ma'am'.

I had heard the name B Corp mentioned in hushed tones.
I got in touch and went to their offices in New York on Wall
Street – the powerhouse of the financial industry. You're
squeezed from both sides of the street by gargantuan

concrete and steel buildings where you can smell the feeding frenzy of business. You know those Attenborough films where a zillion tightly packed minnows are eaten by circling dolphins, who are eaten by circling sharks, who end up being gulped in one mouthful by monstrous blue whales? That's what this place is like. Sitting peacefully in the midst is B Corp. I met Bart Houlahan. We found out we went to the same high school: Evanston Township High School. I asked if we'd dated, as I have very little memory of my early years.

Not only did we not but we hung in diametrically opposite gangs. He was a jock – smart, handsome, football hero – and I was from the buck-toothed loser team, so our paths never crossed. Then we competed over which coffee shops we worked in. I was a waitress at The Huddle where we served omelettes with hair in them. (Most of it mine.) He was a waiter in a really cool place where everyone hung out. (Of course.)

He told me his story. When he left college, he went straight to a financial job in the city. It dawned on him that in order to be in that world, you had to be a touch immoral. He worked a seventy-hour week and had no relationships with colleagues or clients; everything was transactional. The employees screwed anyone in the name of hitting targets, nearly scratching each other's eyes out, fighting for their yearly bonuses. Bart quit and was about to go to Harvard Business School but his friend from school was running an honest-but-small start-up selling basketball footwear. He decided to not go to Harvard but to join his friend, so that he could have a nice life, do good, have healthy relationships and, most importantly, have community. No slouch, he helped make that company a success, growing sales to $250 million in the next eleven years, and the employees shared the profits and all got bonuses. They made their shoes in China but paid workers there a fair wage and made sure they were in a safe environment. They gave 5 per cent of their profits to local charities and urban education. (He is so Patagonia.)

In 2005, he had to sell the firm and found to his horror that, 'when you get to the point where you are ready to sell a company . . . legally, the only thing you are allowed to consider . . . is maximizing shareholder value . . . it felt like I lost a limb to watch all of our commitments to employees, to the environment and to the community be stripped from the company within six weeks of the sale'. His new project became to find a way a company 'could scale up, raise capital, have a liquidity event and still hold on to a mission'. So he co-founded B Lab, a non-profit that sets standards and gives a 'B Corp certificate' that endorses companies that 'want to do good'.

I hadn't realized that, until recently, shareholders could sue a company if it didn't maximize profit; B Lab has created a new law state-by-state across the US and in some countries in Europe and Latin America. Now companies are allowed to have a social or environmental mission written into their charter. So businesses who care about the community and global issues and also are fair to their workers can get a B Corp certificate.

At first no one wanted to be B Corp because it sounded too touchy-feely and they were afraid they'd lose their edge and their money. Now there's an enormous waiting list to get B Corp certified. 'We are at the early stages of one of the most important trends of our lifetime: the growing global movement of people using business as a force for good,' says Bart.

At this point there are 3,260 B Corp businesses around the

world, in seventy-one countries and growing steadily. A few examples are:

The Guardian Media Group (the *Guardian* newspaper in London)

Natura Cosmetics (Brazilian cosmetic company that just bought the Body Shop [now a Certified B Corp] and Avon)

Danone North America (Danone's US subsidiary)

Kickstarter

Participant (formerly Participant Media)

Patagonia (obviously)

Innocent Drinks

Allbirds

Eileen Fisher (clothing)

Ben & Jerry's (owned by Unilever)

Triodos Bank (Amsterdam-based leader of the Global Alliance for Banking on Values)

Each business applying for B Corp certification has to fill in an online assessment regarding their policies: gender and diversity equality, environment and social responsibility. To pass, they have to achieve a certain amount of points and are recertified every three years. Their assessment is made public.

I'm just going to give you the remit of B Corp direct from the horse's mouth because it's so much better than what my mouth can deliver. Here's why the future is getting rosier and kosher-er:

Certified B Corporations are businesses that meet the highest standards of verified social and environmental performance, public transparency, and legal accountability to balance profit and purpose. B Corps are accelerating a global culture shift to redefine success in business and build a more inclusive and sustainable economy.

Society's most challenging problems cannot be solved by government and non-profits alone. By harnessing the power of business, B Corps use profits and growth as a means to a greater end: positive impact for their employees, communities, and the environment. The B Corp community works toward reduced inequality, lower levels of poverty, a healthier environment, stronger communities, and the creation of more high quality jobs with dignity and purpose.

B Corps form a community of leaders and drive a global movement of people using business as a force for good. The values and aspirations of the B Corp community are embedded in the B Corp Declaration of Interdependence.

Unilever

So far, I have been visiting small companies of about 3,000 employees. Some of you more cynical types might be saying to yourselves, 'The small companies can afford to be generous, they only have 3,000 people to worry about.' So just for you guys, I went out to see if there was a corporation that practised this conscious capitalism in the Big-Boy league with more than 100,000 employees. I had heard that Unilever, with 136,000, were doing just that. They're known as the most sustainable company on the map.

Paul Poleman is the ex-CEO of Unilever and famously said: 'Business has to take over where global governments have let us down and now is the moment to do it.' The reason big businesses are more effective at changing things than governments is that they don't have to elect a leader every four years. This means there is no wastage of time and money while your President is only focused on winning the next election. Also, these corporations have far more power and money at their disposal than most governments. Unilever has 2.5 billion consumers a day, present in 98 per cent of households in over 190 countries, generating sales of €52 billion in 2019. They have over 400 brands that include Ben & Jerry's, Dove, Domestos, Omo, Lipton, Breyers, Sunsilk, Surf, Lux, Knorr, etc.

Paul co-founded SDG (Sustainable Development Goals commission) and is co-vice chair of the UN Global Board. I want to quote what he said at a recent SDG meeting because you'll understand why I'd vote for him in any old election.

> 'Two of the biggest challenges that need to be addressed are climate change and inequality . . . I don't want to be responsible for those. Anytime you know that you're polluting and putting carbon in the air, someone else is going to die. Anytime you're wasting food, someone else is going to die . . . We don't need more PhDs, we don't need more people to go to Pluto or Mars to find the answer . . . In the course of history there comes a time when humanity is called upon to shift to a new level of consciousness; it clearly is the moment to do this. You can actually do something to make a difference for generations to come, you can be a real leader by simply bringing humanity back to business. My simple request to you is to live life with purpose.'

We've talked about purpose already but here at Unilever they go in for it in a big way. I was told by the vice president at Unilever that people with a purpose are healthier, can deal with pressure better and, because they have a point to their lives, which is far greater than working at a job, they have a clearer idea of how they want to live and work. To help them find their way they have workshops called 'discover your purpose'. So far 50,000 people who work there have done it and they plan to roll it out to the rest of the 136,000 employees.

If you were going for a job at a certain 'Gordon Gekko' investment bank (I won't mention the name but initials are GS), I heard (maybe it's a rumour) that they give applicants a test that they use for mental patients to find out if they're psychopaths. If the applicant passes the psychopath test, he gets the job. If you want to apply for a job at Unilever, you need skills but they also ask 'What do you want to do in the world?' You may not know but they're looking for people who've thought about it. They said they only want to grow humans there. Paul has put his mouth where his money is.

Day 1 at Four Acres

I was invited to go for a weekend of training at their retreat centre, Four Acres, where I met Tim Munden, Chief Learning Officer, Vice President of HR globally, responsible for well-being. He gave me the history of Unilever (with Power-Point). It was created in 1885 by William Lever (I love this story) who made soap to promote cleanliness and make less work for women. (I don't know what they were doing before – maybe beating clothes against rocks?) He called his product Sunlight Soap and sold over 40 million bars. In 1888 Lever built a village for his employees in the north called Port Sunlight on 150 acres of parkland with more than 900 (now Grade-II listed) buildings, including sports facilities, restaurants, a museum, a gym, art galleries, a theatre, craft activity centres, allotment gardens, football and cricket grounds, swimming pool and community hubs where they could mingle. I keep picturing *The Prisoner*, but there's no big ball chasing anyone and it seems to be a whole village's happy place. When everyone works, plays and cares about each other, we humans are at our best (see my chapter on Communities, I said the same thing). I would have made soap there without any complaints.

In their sustainable living plan these are a list of bullet points; if you read them out and asked people to guess whose plan this was, they might think it was some branch of the UN, not a global corporation.

- Helping more than a billion people take action to improve their health and well-being by 2020.
- Recently committed to ensure 100 per cent of their plastic packaging is fully reusable, recyclable or compostable by 2025.
- Committed to 100 per cent clean energy globally by 2020.
- So far saved over 2,330 tons of greenhouse gases, 120 million tons of water and repurposed 27 million plastic bottles, while donating over $500K to like-minded planet-friendly organizations.
- Made safe drinking water for 55 million people; that's 106 billion litres since 2005.
- 1.85 million women have been empowered through initiatives that develop skills and expand opportunities. (At this point, in management 50 per cent are female.)

Then we have their subsidiary companies' track record . . .

- Lifebuoy, an antibacterial soap, reached 1 billion people through schools, preventing diarrhoea-related death and improving sanitation.
- Domestos, between 2012 and 2017, provided improved sanitation for 16.5 million people in India.
- The tea, PG Tips, Brooke Bond, is helping to tackle social taboos. Their slogan is 'starting a conversation over a cup of tea'. It's India's first transgender brand. They encourage people to bond over a cup of tea and chat about homosexuality and the whole spectrum of LGBTQ (and all the other letters involved). The movement has moved to Russia, Pakistan and Africa.
- Ben & Jerry's, in partnership with the Entrepreneurial Refugee Network, has developed the Ice Cream Entrepreneurs (ICE) Academy, an employment and entrepreneurship programme for refugees. Ninety-six per cent of graduates have obtained employment or started their own business.

What Happens at the 'Discover Your Purpose' Workshop?
Rather than the old business retreats where the suits would hunker down talking 'targets' with squiggly red and green lines on whiteboards (meaning nothing), at the purpose workshop they ask the participants what in their lives had a profound impact, what lights their inner lamps and what do they want to learn about? Also the hardest of all questions, 'Who am I?' I was told that once they figure out their purpose, they can pursue it at work, so life and work become aligned. I asked what their purpose was other than making money? (The elephant in the room.)

Tim invited a few Unilever employees in and asked them to tell me if they'd found their purpose and if so what was it? One example was a woman from communications who said she'd had problems with overeating since she was young so she wanted to help people with the same issues. She works for Dove but decided part of her job was going into schools to teach girls self-esteem. 'Dove #MyBeautyMySay', her project, has been in existence for years. Since 2004 the self-esteem project has reached more than 35 million. She had found her purpose.

Day 2 at Four Acres

Their other plan is to integrate mindfulness throughout the organization, globally. Bit by bit, it's giving their employees insight. If you can't help yourself, you can't help anyone else and that means understanding and being able to calm your rapid-firing mind.

So today, my friend and a great teacher, Louise Chester (who's worked with over 200 organizations) led a group of about thirty people on how to be more mindful, calling it 'the inner game retreat'. When I first met everyone they were like a cluster of job titles. They'd introduce themselves by their role in the company. (Like I'd know what a supply chain manager of Southwest Asia does.) By the end, they were my best friends. The workshop is all about unlearning management and relearning how to be human. Every exercise Louise took us through was punctuated by what she called a 'mindful moment', when we'd stop, become aware of whether our minds had wandered and bring our focus back to the breath. This is how you're able to focus your attention where you want it to be without distraction jerking you around. (This is almost the whole idea of mindfulness.) The point of learning to do these 'moments' is to learn to take these mini breaks to refresh our brains at work.

Daniel Goleman says:

Top performance requires full focus and sustaining focused attention consumes energy – more technically, your brain exhausts its fuel, glucose. Without rest, our brains grow more depleted. The signs of a brain running on empty include, for example, distractedness, irritability, fatigue, and finding yourself checking Facebook . . .

As humans we need to refresh the machine or it will break.

Louise's Lessons for the Survival of the Focused
When the thirty participants arrived, without them knowing what mindfulness is, she had them sit and come into their bodies. Most of us aren't aware we even have one (dragging our brain around all day on this shopping cart made of skin).

She had us pair up with someone nearby and tell them 'who you are'. We had two minutes each. Afterwards, we had to find another partner and again tell them who we were but without repeating the same information we used with the last partner. This kept going with new partners and, running out of our usual schtick, rather than freezing up, people later reported they became more relaxed and connected once they dropped the autopilot banter.

She then gave us all a 'tool for mental effectiveness'. There was a square with quadrants taped on the floor and a title on each section: Mindful, Unmindful, Flow and Creative. We had to stand in the square that defined where we spent most of our time. The Unmindful square was heaving, like peak time on a tube. She then asked which quadrant did we want to spend more time in? What's holding us back from going there? And, finally, what could we do to move into where we wanted to go? I started in the Mindful box because I thought that would prove I was a pro at it but then I realized I had become distracted from the game (my ego had taken over the wheel), so I moved to the Unmindful square.

Louise asked if anyone wanted to share their personal challenges. Many of them 'spilled their beans' emotionally. It may have been the first time they'd spoken from the heart in a safe space and it gave an opportunity to realize that we're all in the same boat, which is usually in some stage of sinking.

At the end of the day, we moved from self-awareness to social awareness. You're no good to anyone if your mind is a mess. Louise punctuated each exercise with a mindfulness practice to reset our inner states. You can only connect to others if your mind is decluttered, non-ruminating and steady, otherwise it's like trying to stand up in that rocking boat. You're no good to anyone and you may just pull everyone on board into the water.

The exercises became about learning to listen (under the words) with compassion and genuine curiosity. Strengthening our ability to discern when to speak and when to shut up; pushing 'pause' to reflect rather than react. Basically, it was about how to be real and how to be human. When you can do all those, you hold the keys to the Kingdom.

If you're leading other people at work, you learn that if you can give someone your full attention, talk to them, human-to-human, they'll trust you, feel safe around you and do the best they can.

What We Learnt Over the Two Days

- That our minds are naturally biased – usually we judge people by who they remind us of, not necessarily who they really are

- What to do when our fear spikes and makes us do stupid things, using mindful exercises to steady it
- How to prioritize what's really important by having a direction that we have decided to move in
- How to reduce multitasking so we don't burn our brains out by focusing on the task in hand
- How to stop always going to worst-case scenario – through mindful retraining of the thought habits
- How to keep our ego in check and to see the bigger picture (this was a big one for me) by seeing and hearing others working with you
- How to get off automatic pilot – to be present – letting go of future or past thinking
- How to have those difficult conversations bringing compassion into the ring

Mindful Moments

We were reminded that our days could be dotted with mindful moments. The idea of the exercise is to see a thought arise and not grab for it. And just by not trying to dissect it or churn it over, watching it begin to dissolve.

Sample Mindful Moments

- Stop
- Notice where you are in the room
- Sense where your body contacts the floor and chair
- Take your focus to your breathing. Notice the minute sensations of inhaling and exhaling and what happens between the in and out breath

- Thoughts will always come and when they do, just be aware, watching them arise and fade, always changing. If you find that hard, give your impulses a label – for example, need to rage at someone, shame, envy, go buy a new car, Bob hates me, etc. You'll notice the list is endless but if you observe the items on it with curiosity and kindness, they won't snare you.

And another . . .

- Count your breaths to ten and then back to one. In-breath, out-breath is one, in-breath, out-breath is two, etc.
- When you notice you're being carried away or lost in thought, take your focus back to the breathing or counting the breaths
- At the end of a few minutes, let go of the exercise and proceed with your life

Eventually, these small mindful moments become a habit. The more moments you take, the more the mind muscles strengthen, to cope with pressure, high emotions, distraction, auto pilot, and become present. There's a useful saying: 'Observe your thoughts as they become actions. Observe your actions as they become habits. Observe your habits, they become who you are and shape your life.' We're the sculptors of our own minds; just by becoming aware of thoughts, without analysing or punishing ourselves for them, they lose their hold and then we begin to reshape our lives.

'If we fail to transform our style of capitalism we will crush humanity out of shape and it will twist itself into tortured forms'
— Charles Dickens

3

Education

Somebody actually made this list for the UK Educational Systems Programme. Let's imagine that while they made it they were thinking these were all fresh, innovative concepts. Even more startling is how far they are from the reality that exists in schools today. Not that they are deliberately flouted – it's just the gap between what you want to do and what actually happens.

Rethinking Education

- We need an education system that excites and stimulates children. (Duh.)
- One size does not fit all. We need a system that enables all children to thrive in their own way, recognizing that young people are individuals with different talents and dreams. (Duh.)
- We must support young people in discovering what they enjoy and are good at – and who they want to be in life. And we must encourage and support teachers and schools in responding to these different needs. Young people will learn if they see learning as important, meaningful and worthwhile. (Duh.)
- Education should be about instilling a sense of wonder and a love of learning. (Duh Duh.)

My Story

My education was way below sea level; nothing stuck on the billboard of my brain but luckily I had the know-how to cheat. For a history test, I wrote the entire 'Declaration of Independence' on my thighs. The only thing that kept me from acing it was that I'd sweated away the details. My head under my skirt, I read, 'All men are created . . .' It was a blur, who knew what they were created for? It was written by Thomas . . . someone (there was only a smudge). People have the rights to 'life, liberty and dslkdjfdsd' (couldn't decipher anything).

During my following years in school, I lost hope, as did my parents, when I found myself in the 'slow' class with students who were all short of a few marbles. I didn't have one of those teachers who saw potential greatness in me; even my typing teacher thought I was 'slow' and she added a note in the report to my mother that she thought I had criminal tendencies. Where she came up with this, I do not know. I once threw up into my electric typewriter which could possibly have electrocuted us all. Barf, poof, gone! But no biggie, so what was her problem?

Education did not make me smart but I excelled in learning how to fail, to hustle and to roll with the punches so I snuck into the cracks of possibilities and went where no high achievers would bother to go. For example, I auditioned over seven times to drama schools that couldn't believe the nerve of someone so abysmal showing up so often with such delusional hope in her eyes. Eventually one in Glasgow let me in, having broken them down, and I went for three happy years to learn the English accent I have today (hear Dick Van Dyke in *Mary Poppins*).

Importance of Failure

I have learnt from this research that learning to fail may have originally been a valuable lesson. (I tell myself this daily.) You can only create something unique by experimenting, which means many of your attempts will hit the fan. It's the struggle to get it right (so something has to be wrong) that gives the results depth and meaning. If you get it right the first time, you're probably copying someone else's work who copied someone else's.

Eventually, at some point in your life you'll fail and those of us who flew the flag of failure in school will know exactly how to deal with it; the captain of the football team will at this point go down in flames. You need a strong failure muscle in life because it's waiting for you around every corner, so be prepared.

School syllabuses make us repetitively go over and over again to learn facts; it's a cycle of preparing, testing, preparing, testing. It's been shown that a better way to learn is trying, failing, trying, failing, but this is hard to incorporate in a system that treats failure as something to be ashamed of.

Teachers today are forced to follow a recipe to make cookie-cutter kids with the required ingredients beaten into them. They're under pressure to get those test results even if the kid is driven half-crazy to achieve them. We're now in danger of being served fast-food education, and as much as fast food is depleting our bodies, this fast-food education is depleting our brains.

My Story

The dream of becoming an actress didn't stop at drama school. Equipped with my Dick Van Dyke accent, I decided my next move would be to get into the Royal Shakespeare Company. Those who I told looked at me with great sadness and my parents laughed like drains. But working on pure chutzpah (also a subject they should teach in schools), I got in. I auditioned by playing an insane American (little did they know the speech wasn't from a play, I was just being me - stream of consciousness). No one can play an insane American better than one who is. They tried to get out of casting me by saying I had to be married to someone British to work in the UK. I found a husband within twenty-four hours (poor man didn't know what hit him). So now they had no excuse and I was in, playing bits of seaweed and an ashtray, but God dammit, I was in.

Juliet Stevenson, also a newcomer, played seaweed next to me. (We once laughed so hard while performing, she peed during *The Tempest* - I was a witness.) I continued to play foliage while she went on to play Cleopatra but to me she'll always be a stalk of seaweed.

'Screw Shakespeare,' I thought, 'I'll write my own shows,' and then I forced Alan Rickman (a fellow member) to direct them. He told me, gently, to avoid acting in the future, that it was not my forte but that I should consider writing comedy. My friends today say there are two big questions in their lives that they know will never be answered. Who shot Kennedy? And how did I get into the RSC? The answer is that it's all done by acknowledging that you may suck at what you're doing but to just steer straight ahead like a deranged arrow to your goal and if you fail, you fail, 'But screw your courage to the sticking place and we'll not fail,' as Lady Macbeth advised. I want to have written on my tombstone, 'At least she tried.'

What's Not Working?

First, let me discuss what's not working in education today and then, as the book promises, what does work.

Some of the questions we have at the moment are the following: Why are so many children burning out from the pressures at school? Why doesn't it prepare them for the reality that's going to smack them in the face when they leave? Why do many leave with an embedded sense of failure before they even have a chance to fail? Why after all these thousands of years haven't we come up with a more inspired and less boring way to teach? Why do we have a system that divides learning into specific subjects that we're force-fed and then required to regurgitate? And, after all that heaving, why doesn't it land us a job?

Today's educational curriculum is based on Victorian manufacturing factory systems developed over a century ago. Kids are put on a learning conveyor belt, then sorted, packaged and labelled according to how their intelligence is measured, and boxed off to the next institution or job (if they're lucky). As someone once said, 'We aren't educating our children, we're domesticating them.'

In the next thirty years, more people will be graduating school than ever so we better come up with some ideas fast. How do we teach our kids anything in an age where their attention has been taken hostage by tech? It's known as 'capturing eyeballs' (a tagline for target marketing). Education needs to somehow figure out how to capture their eyeballs back.

Who is Smart Any More?

We need to rethink what defines someone as smart these days, because we may have got that one wrong. Those with the highest grades and test scores, who then get the top-dog jobs, may know how to turn a profit for a company but they are also equipped with the tools to rob the bank. And some of them arrogantly think they deserve to rob it too. So success at school doesn't guarantee honesty or even sanity. In my opinion, the more powerful you are, the more depleted you may be of human qualities i.e. noticing anyone is alive other than yourself. It's like, again only my opinion, there are very few good-looking people who are also funny. There's a price to pay for certain gifts. Smart also doesn't describe those old-school, puffed-up twats who don't even realize they have spittle dripping down their chin as they smugly spit the details at you of what was the tipple of choice of General Spitoon during the War of the Hardheads in 1458 (I missed a lot in school). We now have to redefine what clever means because, so far, who we called the smartest might just have been having a smidgeon of Asperger's.

Before you think that it's not the schools' fault that some kids can't learn anything, that these kids are born incapable, let me make one thing clear – as Alex Beard titled his book on education (my bible for this chapter), children are all 'Natural Born Learners'.

Early Learning

As far back as 1890, William James, philosopher and psychologist, was saying that babies come into the world as pattern makers. Even in utero, babies are already picking up sounds and trying to find similarities or dissonances. Evolution did its usual 'survival at all costs' thing by preparing them with a skill set to enable them to read clues by picking up information from the environment. Other animals are born with claws, fangs and the means to spurt poison, they don't need to study these, it's instinctive. But for human babies (born with no weaponry up their sleeves), reading faces, picking up emotions and copying what they see is how they learn. When babies see a smile, they feel that whoosh of happiness, whether they're in Panga Panga or Punta de la Gusta. We all need someone to reflect back to. If a baby has no one to mimic, it won't know how to feel emotions or navigate the world and after about a year of not connecting facially and physically to someone, research shows it probably won't survive. The shared attention between baby and parent or caregiver is where conscious learning begins; not just the exchange of words, but the reciprocal feelings. So anyone who can speak and feel has the ability to learn because that's what got them this far.

We come out of the womb like Sherlock Holmes trying to crack the world around us. Everything is intriguing and we want to know what it is, how it works and mostly what it tastes like. (This is why almost everything is shoved into the mouth for investigation first.) It's all a surprise and what motivates us to keep learning is the reward of love and approval we receive in our parents' eyes whenever we guess a colour correctly or give the right name to something. (I know the day my parents stopped smiling at me was when I said 'hat' and pointed to an umbrella.)

So a child isn't born to obey, they are born to explore. They come equipped with a wide-open mind, zapping with all the curiosity in the cosmos and potential to create anything. For the next couple of decades they learn to shrink-wrap themselves into a pre-packaged perfect prototype of a 'student', meaning they function from the neck up, their body only there to move them to the next class.

Whatever grade we get, we forget that it's just a letter for God's sake, not a genetic mutation. You might live your whole life drowning in low self-esteem just because you didn't spell 'catipilar' right even though you might be great at drawing the caterpillar, making music about it, dancing like one, but not being able to spell it means you're a bit of a failure.

This is why kids now suffer higher rates of depression, panic disorders, high anxiety, ADHD, ADD and cutting (that's a new one – it didn't exist in my day). The world is hard enough, couldn't we give kids a break? Allow them to have fun during these years without having to prove how smart they are and feel like failures when they fail? Never again in their lives will they have the ability to just play, without having to prove themselves worthy of being alive by coming home with an 'A'.

After all, you only learn when something lights up the curiosity section of your brain. This is why, at age fifty-seven, I lit up and went to Oxford. My parents would spin in their graves in disbelief. Anyway, you get my point, that my life was lived by the skin of my teeth. (I don't know what that expression means but I'm using it.)

I'm aware of how lucky I am and how lucky my kids are that I made enough to send them to good schools. I'm also aware that some parents either can't get their kids into a decent school or really couldn't care less (which makes it clear to the kid that she's not worth it, so she gives up).

In my hood, the parents are in a white-hot fury of ambition; they tear their hair out if their kid gets below a 'C', as in their opinion it stands for loser. (C was my best grade – I always think a letter C looks like someone hunkered over a toilet, throwing up.) Anyway, they have their offspring tutored up the wahzoo. Actually, from the moment the head crowns in the cervix, they want the baby tested to get them into the 'best' school and then the 'best' next school and then the 'best' university . . . and the rejects peel off like burning parts of a rocket that are only holding it back. What destroys a kid's mind faster than a speeding bullet is a parent who pushes. Twenty years later, these same uber-ambitious mothers now ask if I know of a good rehab? The harder the kids were pushed, the harder the drugs they become hooked on.

Humans learn best when they feel someone cares about them, not for their intelligence, looks or talent but for who they are. This is not how education in school works today so kids are burning out faster than they ever did before; one in three now suffers from some kind of mental health problem. The good news is coming, which I'll reveal later in the chapter, but at this stage, just to put everything in context, I'd like to give you my version of the history of education – it's completely accurate, I just took out the boring bits of which there were many.

The History of Education

In the Beginning . . .

There was no formal education for thousands of years, when we were apes, it was recess all the time. Those were the days. Only when we turned into humanoids did we start to have lessons. Hunters taught young boys to hunt, gatherers taught the fine art of gathering to the girls – which was not as fun. The good news was that the kids learnt by imitation, not repetition, it was all outdoors and there were no grades. Playtime was when we weren't hunting or gathering, and if you were eaten, you were eaten (shit happens), you weren't trained to be paranoid by your parents. Not like today where you get into trouble with social services if you let your kid run loose. You can't get away with saying, 'Sorry, officer, I was just teaching Zack to hunt.' Anyway, no one was forced to be exceptional. Obviously, there were some naturally bright, talented cave people. Maybe the one who started etching horses on the cave walls in France won the equivalent of what the Turner Prize is today.

Around 2.5 million years ago, stone tools were discovered in Ethiopia, which suggests that education was no longer monkey see, monkey do, but someone was writing or drawing things that could be handed down from generation to generation, sharing knowledge on everything from how to skin something and make it into a hat to general knowledge on how to survive. It couldn't have been that informative because Homo sapiens (meaning 'wise human beings') did not emerge from Africa until around 200,000 years ago. It took them all that time to grow a cerebrum to a decent size and develop vocal apparatus so they could speak. If the instructions were that good, don't you think they would have evolved faster than that? (Let's just say that manual did not become number one on the hominid bestseller list.)

A stone tablet found in Mesopotamia and dating from 2000 BC provides a glimpse into what early schooling looked like:

- The student took a packed lunch to school
- His subjects included Sumerian arithmetic and book-keeping
- The 'school father' (teacher), the school porter and superintendent would be in charge of discipline (beating)
- These first schools in Babylon were referred to as 'tablet houses'

Then, in Classical times, the whole learning system was reinvented. The Greek word for school was *skhole* and meant 'lecture house'. What they read at *skhole* was really boring; it was like reading the Yellow Pages and they also mainly learnt about accounts.

The First Thousand Years of Modern Education

When Plato's Academy and Aristotle's Lyceum came along, the young students in Athens learnt the 3Rs followed by apprenticeship for a trade (if you were a pleb), while the patrician elite learnt drawing, sculpture, rhetoric (winning arguments), maths, geography, natural history, politics and logic; pretty much what you would get taught at Eton today.

Socrates didn't believe you could learn anything by writing it down so he invented the process of learning through asking questions. Like a game show minus the buzzer, it was all about face-to-face interaction and the purpose was to ask questions like, 'The unexamined life is okay for cows but not for us. Discuss.' He put philosophy on the map (it means love of wisdom) but was eventually put to death for asking too many questions, so it did him no favours.

Socrates' general theories continued through the rest of BC times. We are told that Jesus was praised for asking such challenging questions at his bar mitzvah. (I'm not sure it was there but he was Jewish so he probably had one – not a big fancy one but in the stable or something.)

After that for about 500 years the only learning was in monasteries where lessons were delivered in Latin. Good luck if you didn't speak it. Here, students learnt grammar, rhetoric and logic. I would have flunked out.

Later, Martin Luther (1483–1546, German priest who started the Protestant Reformation) got it in his head, before he lost it, that salvation depended on each person being able to read the scriptures in their own language, so at least they dropped the Latin.

When the fall of the monasteries occurred, the fall of education for anyone other than the rich came too; it then cost a fortune and it was mostly private tutoring (the birth of hot-housing). Poor people just learnt how to be poor over and over again until they understood how poor they really were.

Meanwhile in America

In the US in the mid seventeenth century, Massachusetts became the first colony to mandate schooling to keep the kids obedient by training them to be good Puritans. They learnt to read from a primer known as the 'Little Bible of New England', which had short rhymes to help kids learn the alphabet, beginning with 'A. In Adam's fall, we sinned all.' It went through the whole alphabet, each letter with a saying about the Lord, ending with Z for Zacchaeus, 'He did climb the tree, his Lord to see.' All the lessons were to instil fear of God and the wrath of adults if you faltered. Also the rhymes were shit.

From Factory Fodder to Classroom

In the Industrial Age, kids moved from the bondage of rural poverty to the factory floor. They worked seven days a week, many dying of disease and starvation, and if they did manage to go to school they just learnt the basic numbers and letters; the duller the subjects taught in schools, the better to numb their minds. Then, in 1883, England passed laws limiting child labour, saying that children couldn't work under the age of nine and restricting weekly work hours to forty-eight for ten- to twelve-year-olds and sixty-nine for thirteen- to seventeen-year-olds. Imagine today, telling your kid they'd have to work even for ten minutes; they'd take you to court.

In the nineteenth and twentieth centuries, as industry became automated, the need for child labour declined in parts of the world. Childhood as a concept was invented at this point (before that, kids were considered mini adults) so this was when we got those paintings of a 'wittle' girly sucking her thumb with cutesy blonde curls, a teardrop in her eye, holding a kitten. It may come as a surprise that these adorable images of children didn't stop the Victorians from continuing to beat them senseless. Their justification for this was that as they were born evil, it was necessary to discipline them to keep them obedient. This clearly attracted people of a sadistic nature to become school teachers. One master in Germany kept records of the floggings he did in fifty years of teaching: 911,527 blows with rod, 124,010 with cane, 136,715 blows with hand and 1,118,800 blows on head. Punishments were understood as being a natural part of the educational process and most people thought play was a waste of time, but they let them out once in a while to let off steam. It turns out recess is important after you've been slammed. Who knew?

Everything stayed pretty much the same. The rich people went to Eton to study talking like a peacock and running the country, and the poor had to study the Bible so they'd know what God could do to them if they tried to step out of line.

Twentieth Century

Scroll on a bit, then bingo, in 1954 the National Union of Teachers in the UK decided that the quarter of a million teachers, free from government or Church interference, could decide what should be taught, how it should be taught and then go teach it.

So by the 1970s, experimental schools were opening, where kids had no rules and studied having sex with everyone, including teachers. Sadly, it didn't work as standards went to pot. Schools were failing to produce kids who could even read and write (there had been too much of an emphasis on finger-painting) and there was an economic downturn, making people nervous that the UK would go down the drain because schools were producing kids with the academic ability of glow-worms.

A few years later, Thatcher came to power and as a result of various complaints and media exposure of failing schools, she took out her whip and put a halt to free-fall education. It seemed we didn't need people majoring in pottery. And that was the birth of today's highly controlled National Curriculum where all children were taught maths, English, science, a foreign language, history, geography and technology, and tests were introduced based on attainment targets, at ages seven, eleven and fourteen. (What do you know at seven, besides spitting at people? That was my major then.)

The final phase was when we invented Ofsted and now teachers were no longer considered to be in the same professional league as doctors or lawyers and started being examined and scrutinized by inspectors on what and how to teach. Boxes had to be ticked and targets reached; the kids went into their rooms and put on headphones.

Where We Are Today

So that's how we got to where we are. Now, please don't burn me at the stake for what I'm going to say, it's just my opinion. Though these subjects are fascinating and very important for exercising our brains, they will not ensure a job in the future; they say that in thirty years' time, 80 per cent of today's eight-year-olds will have jobs that haven't even been invented yet. Knowing that Churchill liked to play miniature golf on days off or King Leo the Lionheart had a stutter will not get you work in 2030. In the meantime, computers can do the maths, spellcheck can do the spelling, a USB stick can hold memory and Wikipedia knows everything.

My suggestion would be to start giving kids degrees in 'people skills', which is something I doubt any computer will ever accomplish, mainly because the coders who do the coding can't code it into the programs because most of them have no idea what people skills are. Hopefully, the CEOs in the future will be there because they got 'A's in Empathy.

Something to feel good about, though, is that teachers are very safe from being replaced by robots. When it comes to classroom management, I don't know how an avatar could stop the back row using biros as blowpipes and covering the ceiling with screws of paper.*

League Tables and Why They're Shit

Not only are the kids set against each other at school like chickens in a cockfight, now schools, thanks to the league tables, are ranked against each other to be the 'best', forcing head teachers into the business of chasing results like the CEO from a bank. The current system is making teachers 'teach to the test' so that lessons are focused on getting

---

* Post-Covid, there is far more virtual and online teaching, but you still need a teacher to do it. Homeschooling is most parents' idea of hell.

the kids to swallow and then spew out the syllabus. Henceforth to be known as the 'swallow 'n' spew' model.

Then there is the big scary monster called PISA – Programme for International Student Assessment – that is an international survey which evaluates education systems worldwide by testing fifteen-year-old students. Every three years, students in over ninety countries are tested on reading, maths and science. So, now it's not just a cockfight between UK schools, it has become a worldwide competition. The UK has flopped over the years. Guess who's in front? China, Singapore and Japan.

The highest-performing schools in the world are in Shanghai. These countries push their kids into whatever generates the most capital, putting the economy first, rather than the children. Guess what's sacrificed? Well-being, a moral code, personal development, emotional intelligence, improvement of relationships, communication – all tools for a better life.

China

I'm aware that my international readership might be feeling left out so to make them feel included, I went to the East – my books are translated into Chinese, it's the least I can do. Coincidentally, I'd been invited to do a talk at a school in Shanghai, which was a branch of Wellington College UK where Sir Anthony Seldon was the headmaster for twenty years. He's convinced that truly happy people are made, not born, and so created his own curriculum which included mindfulness; the school's academic results shot through the roof. He identifies five really important things he has learnt in life:

• Stop worrying
• Happiness is the opposite of selfishness

- Learn from experience not just university
- Be yourself
- Live by water

I understand all of these except the last one. I was asked to go and give a talk on mindfulness in Shanghai.

11 April 2019

Before going to Wellington, Shanghai, I asked if I could visit a regular Chinese school. I had to send in my 'intentions', which didn't bode well, but then they found out I worked in TV as an entertainer so the gates were thrown open and I was greeted by a smiling staff and a neon sign with my name in lights. As soon as I entered the halls, I noticed there was no noise anywhere. I was told the reason was that everyone gets a number of points called social credit and if anyone misbehaves they deduct points, which will affect their future job opportunities. So no one acts up, and if they do, their peers will report them and gain points for themselves.

I walked into a classroom; none of the students turned around. They sat stiff, facing forward like little numb soldiers with Chinese Miss Trunchbull from *Matilda* at the helm. She was writing mile-long equations on the board, expecting immediate, speeding-bullet answers. I spoke to friendly Trunchbull afterwards who told me maths shapes the brain, knowledge doesn't count, memorization makes muscles as does competition, which results in a better life. You make money, you have success and it guarantees a better partner. (Clearly they marry for maths.) She referred to the humanities – history, language, philosophy – as 'arts', with a curled lip of disdain.

I was told that a thirteen-year-old has the equivalent

intelligence of a UK university student and that Chinese parents are famous for their tyrannical discipline to 'help' the child at home. Some use various methods of beating which I don't remember finding in my 'How to bring up baby' books. But, boy, does it get results. If the kid gets below 100 per cent it's considered shameful and may call for more beating.

There is no Mr or Mrs Nice Guy, the parents compete ruthlessly with other families for whose kid's smartest and which of their kids sleeps the least. (That's high status here.) Some of the kids stand up in lessons so they don't fall asleep, which would also be considered shameful. There is no time off; after they finish school they have four hours of homework, then many are privately tutored until 2.00 a.m. (Tutors who get the best results can make about $400,000 a year. Parents spend about 70 per cent of their income on education so their kid better hit that 100 per cent.) After all this, some kids are chained to a violin or piano to become maestros at age three then have to get up again at 5.30 a.m. All this happens so the parents don't 'lose face', the biggest taboo of them all.

I asked discreetly if any of the kids suffer from depression or other mental problems. The answer was, 'Very little.' I was told there is suicide, but no depression, which is good.

If they do show signs of a 'problem', including dyslexia, they may be asked to leave school for a year and are taken to the country. Then, I was told, some are, strangely, never heard of again. (I think this has always been an excellent cure, especially for dyslexia.) However, if a kid thinks he needs help (and this is shameful), he goes to the school counsellor. I went to meet her in a small room where she showed me her technique for kids with 'concentration' problems. In the middle of the room there was a sandbox filled with white sand. Shelves along the walls were filled with miniature toy figures: housewives, soldiers, clowns, ballet dancers along with plastic trees, tiny furniture, model cars, etc. The kid with the 'concentration' problem is asked to put whatever they want on the sand. I asked why and the counsellor told me she had no idea. But she assured me, if the sand therapy doesn't help there are other methods. I was taken down the hall and proudly shown a red padded room where the kids can hurl themselves around and bang off the walls to let off steam. There are life-sized blow-up figures which they can club till bursting. (I'm guessing they represent parents or teachers.)

Suddenly, hideous carnival music was pumped into the airwaves to eardrum-shattering volume. This marks the time when all the students stop what they're doing and do exercises for the eyes. In circling movements, they massage their cheekbones and the sides of the head to improve their eyesight. Many of the kids wear glasses from straining their eyes through the long hours of study and this improves their sight. These same kids who are maths geniuses think the rubbing of the face cures defective eyesight. I didn't question it out loud. I left with the teachers waving me farewell as the kids still sat riveted to their seats, chanting numbers like automatons.

Well, there you have it, the highest grade results in the universe making China the richest country in the world and no one has any mental problems. Problem solved.

Oh, did I mention China and Korea (another hothouse of schooling and where my book is sold) have the highest suicide rate among thirteen- to twenty-four-year-old girls in developed nations and the boys aren't far behind.

12 April 2019

I was introduced to Ewan, head teacher from Wellington College, who couldn't have been more loving. Ewan loved *Girls on Top* (my first TV show) so he made sure my every whim was fulfilled. I had the day off and he had to teach so he gave me Yvette as a guide to show me the sights of Shanghai.

We didn't understand each other right off the bat. Yvette told me she was my 'Urine' and I should call her that. I said maybe not. A few days later we figured it out, she was saying she was my 'Ewan' for the day. At one point, I told her I had gum and she blanched. She whispered, 'You can't have gum in China, it's against the law.' I figured it's that litter law again where you can't deface the sidewalks. I asked her if she wanted some, she nearly fainted. She told me they frisk you in the metro and if they find it on you, you're arrested. I asked her if anyone is allowed gum? She told me only the police for security reasons. I told her I'm going to use it anyway because what's the worst that can happen? She said, 'You could shoot people,' to which I asked, 'By spitting gum at them?' Gradually it dawned on us both she was talking about guns. We bonded after that.

She took me to see some of the more unusual sights of Shanghai. Each Sunday, in People's Park, hundreds of parents sit behind umbrellas which have a sheet of paper pinned on them. The paper gives information about the son or daughter, advertising them for potential marriage. (I guess it's their version of Tinder – though they're supposed to be so technically advanced and here they're using umbrellas to deliver information. See what I mean, how confusing these people are?) So there they are, the parents perched on little boxes, behind their parasols, pimping the kids.

Yvette translated some of their CVs:

'Single daughter of Ning, height 1.68 metres. Worked at Goldman Sachs for two years; now chief engineer at Apple looking for boyfriend. Nianha is honest, self-motivated, wants boy over number 10,000 in Shanghai.' (There is a quaint old system here in Shanghai where they number you in order of how smart you are. In a city of 24 million, 10,000 isn't chopped liver.)

Another one said, 'Unmarried man born 1989, height 1.70 metres, graduated in finance, stock analyst, can buy house, looking for kind lady as companion.' (I almost answered that one.)

13 April 2019

It's my first day at Wellington College and it's a whole differ-ent barrel of fish to the first school I saw. You hear laughter, kids are playing football outside, teachers are smiling.

I was shown to a classroom where I would be doing a talk on mindfulness and found there were no children, only Chin-ese parents. When I got to a point about stress, everybody's face went blank. I asked if the translator spoke English, thinking it was her fault, but she explained to me that people in China don't have stress. I wondered why I had been brought here in the first place. I asked how they reacted to being pumped with bad news about wars, crime, disaster – didn't it frighten them? She told me that there's no bad news on TV or digitally because it's censored so they only hear news of how wonderful China is and that the rest of the world is a cesspit of corruption and that they should consider themselves lucky to be there. She explained that even if they did feel something like stress, they would lose face. I had to remind myself that though I was at a liberal school, this stuff is deeply ingrained. I politely asked if there was a biology teacher in the house, and if there was, did these kids ever learn about the damage cortisol does to the brain from the pressure of learning even while they're saving their faces? There was a biology teacher who raised his hand but looked blank. (I think 'blank' is the 'in' look in China.) When I asked what he taught the kids, I swear he said, 'Polar bears,' but maybe it was lost in translation.

Later, when I met the children, I asked them how they defined happiness. A boy who shone with intelligence told me he equated happiness with money and when I asked how he pictured happiness, he said a pool with gold coins at the bottom. I thought, now I'm really wasting my time.

In the afternoon I did my show, *Frazzled*, in the theatre attended by parents and teachers. At a point in the show I talk about how I was a great failure at school because I thought out of the box when those around me didn't even know there was a box. Then I say, 'And what happened to all those girls who got straight "A"s and were cheerleaders and everyone expected them to do so well? Well, now they're all crack whores.' The woman who was translating just ground to a halt, no idea what it meant, the parents went blanker than any blank I'd ever seen but the teachers laughed and applauded. A bizarre experience.

Because some of these kids (mainly those with a Western parent) will go to university in the US or Europe, they are also offered classes in emotional intelligence. I watched a class where the students learnt how to read each other's emotional state by noting the tone of voice, posture and word choice. They learnt how to understand 'below the words' by listening with their 'whole body' as they call it. They practised how to hold back on instant gratification, to pause before reacting and to notice their own biases before responding. There's an exercise I watched them do to help them tolerate uncomfortable feelings of boredom, confusion and bewilderment.

When they have to get their heads down for the pressure of academic courses, they've learnt to get their minds cool and collected to take in information and consolidate it with ease. What an irony that in China they're teaching kids empathy. (Mao would spin in his grave.) As I said before, I think social skills will be the gold standard in the future and Wellington is ahead of the game.

Here, when they teach maths, it's not dry theory, it's taught with an application in mind. Rather than chant numbers, the kids learn how to make solar panels which they send to places like Cambodia for people without electricity or they make seismographs out of cardboard to detect earthquakes or a robot for the purpose of delivering medicine. They have a website called solarbuddy.com where the students build tech (drones, robots, programs, apps) for anything that's needed anywhere in the world. So here, in the land of the red dragon, there are signs of green shoots.

The Bad News for Tech in Education

There seems to be some evidence around that says passive screen-sucking is not just unhelpful to children's learning, but could set back their development. As always, I'm not knocking tech but we need to keep our fingers on the pulse to make sure we're still pumping blood not electricity. With too much screen time the 'white matter' in their brains depletes, impacting numeracy and language skills. 'Babies require face-to-face interaction to learn,' says Dr Vic Strasburger, professor and spokesperson for the American Academy of Paediatrics. 'The watching probably interferes with the crucial wiring being laid down in their brains during early development.' Even if they're watching an educational programme, like *Sesame Street*, it delays language development. I'm so sorry, Big Bird, I loved you, I had no idea you were stunting my mental growth.

Dr Vic also says that children's videos are causing a generation of overstimulated kids. People assume that stimulation is good, so the more the better, but it's not true, there is such a thing as overstimulation. The more television children watch, the shorter their attention spans later in life. 'Their minds come to expect a high level of stimulation, and view that as normal, and by comparison, reality is boring.' For those who want to know what the screen-time limit is for them to allow their kids, here are the guidelines.

The ideal number of hours on screen for kids aged two to five is up to an hour a day. For teens it's up to about two hours a day. Good luck getting them off. If anyone has any ideas about how it's done, please write to me.

Using a computer to help you with a problem or to find information actually makes the brain lazy and deskills you in the long term. When the brain can take a shortcut, it does, but in doing so it fails to lay down the cognitive architecture needed to deepen intelligence. Proof of this is the overuse of the satnav. Many of us no longer know where we live without it. We have lost the ability to find our way home.

The Good News

However, green shoot-wise, tech can democratize opportunities for learning globally at a much lower cost than formal, classroom-based learning, often offering it for free for those unable to pay. If a kid has access to a smart device and a Wi-Fi signal, even in the remotest village in Africa or some sliver of an island in the Pacific, they can learn anything. Developing countries don't want third-rate schools so the students are better off with remote course providers.

I don't know if you've looked at what's available online but even at the universities you could never get into in real life, you can take a course remotely. You can no longer get away with saying, 'I missed the bus.' The greatest of all professors are a click away and if you find one boring, just click another. Here are some examples of what's out there:

- Udemy gives a choice of 100,000 video courses to choose from; if a university did that it would have to be the size of Albania.
- Coursera college education is low cost and is being taught by professors from Princeton, Johns Hopkins and Stanford.
- Futurelearn is completely free, offering courses in business, creative arts, law, health, politics, science and digital skills.
- Other sites give you access to Harvard, Yale, MIT, Oxford, Cambridge, and there's even an ITunes University. (You probably just hum along with classes.)

In all the courses, you have the chance to interact and chat with instructors, unlike in real life where they will never in a million years have time to see you personally. There's also interaction with fellow students so you aren't learning in a bubble. You can learn on planes, trains and automobiles with 'real-time interactivity'. You can study in the bathtub, but if you do, I'd shut off the interactive button.

Here's a bonus: rather than online dating, which may still be weird for some, you can hook up with someone in your class who has similar interests. You can pretend you're studying together and then make your move. It may be difficult if one of you is in Siberia and the other in Abu Dhabi, but it's worth a try.

A study in 2018 showed 85 per cent of students who had previously enrolled in face-to-face courses and then switched to online courses felt that the online experience was the same or better than the classroom. So you can get any degree, in anything, just sitting at home in your underwear.*

Even More Good News

I met Lee Daley at TEDTalks, co-founder of an emerging technology called Hello Genius. He calls it a 'platform for outlier kids' aged three to nine years old. This covers kids with learning disabilities to kids who are unique and don't fit in the conventional educational system. The individual machine learning and AI encourages kids who think differently; it caters to those who think out of the box.

When using Hello Genius, they 'embark on a self-guided exploration through a treasure trove of knowledge'. Their imagination leads the programme, rather than being forced through what he describes as the 'cookie cutter' education system. By the way, Ken Robinson is on their board, who is deeply opposed to cookie-cutter teaching.

Also, Daley says, when you tell a student to 'pay attention' and they don't, usually there's a reason behind it. Probably, you're not capturing their attention, that's why they're not paying it. Most of us adults don't even know where our attention is from moment to moment, so how would a kid? Attention has to be captured first and then trained. This programme follows the attention of the learner. For example,

* Post-lockdown, this is rather obvious, with online lessons being the new norm.

the kid types in 'dinosaur' and images of hundreds of dinosaurs come up on the screen. They're then encouraged to
zoom in to the one which takes their interest. Choices come
up about things you might want to learn about the dinosaur.
What's their favourite food? Who do they like to kill and
how? When did they die out? Etc. Whatever the kid taps in
leads to more choices. Let's say, they want to watch a ptero-
dactyl fly and that ignites their curiosity about how
aeroplanes fly, so they tap a button to watch a video of aeroplanes, which may make them wonder how wind works and
with another tap an expert tells them about meteorological
reasons for gales. You get the picture? They can choose what
excites them, through their minds and fingers. Whenever
they tap a choice, another world opens up. Curiosity rules.

This is using tech as a teacher to widen their minds. The
data also allows parents to get an insight into what their
child is really stimulated by. If they see their daughter is
interested in aerodynamics, get her a toy rocket and not
some cliché pink doll they think she'd like. Or if the boy has
a penchant for making tutus, give him the doll. Isn't this an
exciting development?

And Now For the Really Really Good News: REAch2

I visited a state school in the UK that is beyond a green shoot,
it's a fully thriving tree.

REAch2 is a radically new type of school, a type of school
that I wish I'd gone to. There are two primary schools: Tidemill Academy in Deptford, London, and Garden City Academy
in Letchworth, Hertfordshire. Both are part of an Academy
Trust run by a state-funded charity. It started with a few schools
and now is the biggest school trust in the country, serving over
sixty schools – that's about 20,000 students. It's partnered with

Mindfulness in Schools. At the start, 17 per cent were considered 'good' by Ofsted standards; now the figure is 82 per cent, which is in the top 10 per cent in the UK, with their SATs results 23 per cent above national average. Half the kids come from a 'deprived' background (free school meals). A further twenty-two REAch2 schools are going to be opened in the next few years. The idea, besides teaching them formal education, is to grow these kids into great human beings; discovering who they are, what their responsibility is to the world and how to show compassion to themselves and others.

REAch2 promises to give kids eleven positive experiences before they turn eleven. It's the kids' choice what those are: to visit a foreign country, cook meals from vegetables they grew themselves, climb a mountain, sleep under the stars, paddle down a river; things they could never do in their normal lives. They are also challenged to do ten good deeds in ten days.

I went to look around Letchworth Garden City Academy. There was a notice I passed that said, 'Big feelings are not to be ashamed about but they may stop us from doing what we want in life and affect our mental health. If your feelings are too big to cope with on your own, you can speak to Leila at Place to Talk in room 130.'

Other signs around the school said:

'Your background has nothing to do with your achievement.'

'I am a good person, even if I am angry. I can calm myself down. I'm in control.'

'I believe in myself. I can work hard. I can accomplish anything I set my mind to.'

'Kindness is my superpower.'

'I am smart. I am special. I can do hard things.'

'Right now. Think of things to be thankful for.'

I met a group of nine-year-olds who told me their names and then how they felt; they call it 'checking in'. Most told me they were nervous meeting an outsider. (My own kids never told me how they felt outside of a grunt.) They study the brain to learn what happens inside themselves when their brain gets aroused and when it's calm. The teacher had them do an exercise where they go around the circle saying what was special about themselves. A little overweight boy said that kids used to tease him but he's learnt to be kind to him-self and therefore be kind to others. If they started bullying him he used to get into fights; now he walks away and later writes down what the bully might have been thinking and feeling – it wasn't about him after all.

Another exercise they did is called the 'train of love' where they go in a circle, telling the person to their right what they like most about them. They said things like 'being there for me' and 'letting me tell my secrets to you'; the kid next to me said to me, 'Thank you for helping kids and coming to see us today.' This is a tribe if ever there was one. One kid talked about how his dad was stuck like a marble in a bottle and he wanted to help him get out. The children now tell me they're teaching their parents to focus on their breathing when they feel they're about to blow; their parents are shouting less.

After school, the kids have about thirty clubs to choose from as an alternative to going home for video games.

They all are assigned a 'buddy' to bond with, always pair-ing an older student with a younger one, helping each other with problems and becoming like a little family, which they might not have at home. They practise listening to each other mindfully, giving each other their full attention so they both 'feel heard'.

To teach them to deal with tough situations and learn to self-reflect, they're given a workbook. On the first page is an exercise which they fill in.

You have made a choice to do something and that means you need to stop and think about the following things:

What did I choose to do?
Why did I make this choice?
Who did my choices affect?
How did this affect them and make them feel?

By making this choice, I was not showing . . . . Check which one applies:

Respect
Resilience
Enthusiasm
Curiosity
Appreciation
Empathy

Have I apologized to the people I affected?
Do I think this has helped?
What could I have done instead?
From now on I will . . . .

Then there's a drawing of a boy crying, with questions:

What words can you see in the boy's tears?
What are these tears representing?

What would your tears say?
Did the boy build a wall and have you ever put a wall up
so people don't know how you're feeling?
Do you have someone kind in your life?
How can you be someone's kind person?

On my visit to the school in China the kids were like robots, all facing forward, chanting the answers by rote. Here at Letchworth Garden City Academy, as I passed the classroom, the kids all smiled and waved for me to come in.

I went in and each room had a 'regulation zone', which was a place to take 'time out' when they felt overwhelmed. In the space there was a cardboard sheet on the wall coloured red, blue, yellow and green. The kids are allowed to get up and move to the colour zones. Here they choose a colour that helps them identify their feelings. If you can name it, you can tame it. The red zone has the words: furious, frustrated, shocked, frightened, restless, worried, uneasy, etc. Blue has the words: disgusted, mortified, alienated, glum, excluded, drained, alone, bored, tired, etc. The yellow zone has the words: surprised, joyful, hyper, thrilled, inspired, energized, proud, blissful, etc. The green zone has the words: humble, blessed, calm, relieved, relaxed, tranquil, fulfilled, etc. There are also pictures of facial expressions so they can identify their mood. Once they identify their state they use tools to help them get to the green zone. They can write down the answer to the questions: *What were you doing that made you feel in that state? What can help you next time to get to the green or yellow zone?* Once they identify their feelings, if they're in the blue or red zone, they have options. They can listen to calming music on earphones or practise various mindfulness exercises to help them focus on sight, sound, taste and touch. There's a breathing ball to help them become aware of their breathing. When they push the ball in with both hands they breathe out and when they release the ball they breathe in. There's a 'mindfulness jar' filled with water and glitter. When they feel chaotic they shake the jar to reflect their minds. Then they hold it still and watch the glitter settle and imagine this is their mind settling. There's a green snake-like stuffed animal which, when they put it around their necks, they told me, feels like someone is hugging them. There are bubbles which represent their negative thoughts, which they can blow (only a few) and then pop them so they get the idea that thoughts aren't solid, they're as insubstantial as soap bubbles.

They talk about the amount of sleep they need and what happens to their brains when they don't sleep enough. Newborn babies up to three months need fourteen to seventeen hours' sleep, infants from four to eleven months need between twelve and fifteen hours' sleep, toddlers (one to two years) need between eleven and fourteen hours. School-age children from six to thirteen years will need between nine and eleven hours.

They have tools for helping them sleep using a technique from the .b Mindfulness in Schools Project where they do a body scan last thing at night in bed to help them relax from their toes up to the top of their heads. Or by putting a favourite stuffed animal on their stomachs and watching it go up and down, then noticing how the movement slows down when their breathing slows down. Thousands of schools in the UK use the .b curriculum to help kids learn to regulate their stress levels, focus their attention, come into the present and use empathy.

In the afternoon I was taken to the Zen Den in the garden where they learn to plant vegetables, then take them home and cook them for their parents. A little girl told us she never saw a courgette (or zucchini if you're from my land) before or knew lettuce grew in the soil.

Builders, decorators, painters and electricians volunteered from the community to create the Zen Den even though they didn't understand what it was for. The kids were all sitting on cushions where a little girl led us in a mindfulness exercise which she wrote herself.

> Sit comfortably, shoulders relaxed, hands on your lap. Close your eyes if you wish to. Take 3 slow, deep breaths in and out.
> (Pause – count to 17)
> Breath in all that is kind and happy.
> Breath out all that is negative and unwanted.
> (Pause – count to 17)
> Smile into your heart.
> Take a moment and, when you are ready, wiggle your fingers and toes.
> Slowly open your eyes.

Another girl did stretching mindfulness, instructing the kids to stretch to the sky and feel the sensations in their bodies, open their arms, taking in the universe. And then shake all negativity out. At the end she told them all to picture their happy place.

A little boy led a mindfulness sound exercise, telling us to take in all the sounds around us, tune in to them and allow the sounds to come to us. He wanted us to tune in to the rain outside. He said it reminded him of his sadness but then, when it hits the ground, it disperses. He uses the image at home where many members of his family suffer from mental illness so there's always screaming. The teacher told me he used to have violent meltdowns, once punched through a glass door, but now he walks away and does the breathing ball.

At the end of the day the whole school, all 600 of them, gathered in an assembly and sang out, glowing with happiness, the song 'A Million Miles'. Afterwards, they gave me a 'thank you' card that read: 'Dear Ruby, many, many thanks. You wonderful delighter. Your presence made our day happier and brighter. From all the children and staff at Garden City Academy.' With every student's fingerprints on the front. Well, no matter how strong my medication was, I had to cry even though I don't like that song.

How We Should Measure Educational Success

All good learning takes place when you are either passionate about the subject or you're having fun. In a study on how to measure success, those who are naturally proficient at a subject have a highly developed sense of play. Doing something over and over can make you proficient but won't help you produce something original. As Adam Grant (brilliant organizational psychologist) said, 'Practice makes perfect but can't make new.'

In the book *Natural Born Learners*, Alex Beard talks about this and says that now neuroscience is mapping our brains and finding that inspiration is only achieved when you're not focused. Creativity comes out of associative thinking, not from depth but breadth of knowledge. My greatest ideas come to me in the shower, so I have to run out naked to type my gem. Alex quotes Einstein, who said, 'The greatest scientists are artists too,' and that 'the theory of relativity came to me by intuition' (I bet he was in the shower).

In Finland they have taken this to a whole new level and are achieving high results in a breakthrough new way. So off I went to discover how and why.

Finland, the Hope for the Future: A Country of Green Shoots

As a birthday present, my son Max said he'd take me on a holiday of my choice. I asked for Finland because it's recently been the 'It Girl' of travel. Out of nowhere, suddenly, everyone wants to go to Finland, so I had to go. I'd never even used the word 'Finland' before and suddenly I was obsessed, picturing reindeers jingling everywhere you look and taking dog sleds to local markets which are 'Christmassy' all year round, with everyone living in saunas, drinking glögg (this is the power of good branding). It turns out it's not exactly what it says on the label. First of all, the saunas: as you enter what could be a wooden outdoor loo, you see horrible igloos of human flesh sizzling by a bowlful of burning coals. Helsinki itself is what I like to call 'late Soviet bloc, early gulag': big concrete slabs of buildings with tiny tinted windows for spying, housing dead shopping malls selling cheap clothes and herring. And then suddenly the depression architecture stops and you walk straight into a forest. Not even a park, it's a forest with lakes in the middle. There it is, like Narnia, from concrete to a carpet of greenery in one step. There are forests everywhere in this city, all where you least expect them. So we kayaked across a lake and hit a sidewalk where our mode of travel was electric scooters, dodging street cars on cobbled streets so wobbly that my liver fell out. There are 5.5 million people in the whole country so you have no fear of crashing into anyone because they don't exist. Basically, Finland is not charming but the good news is it costs a fortune.

I have to be honest, there is one building that sucked the oxygen out of me, it was so spectacular and unexpected: the Oodi Helsinki Library, 17,250 metres of undulating waves made of curved Finnish spruce wrapped by curved glass. Everything in here is free for the locals: 3D printers, screening rooms, VR equipment, robot librarians (who don't just tell you to 'shut up' – you can play with them), cubbyhole womb rooms lined with orange leather seating to meditate in (picture sitting inside a pumpkin). I won't go on but it's worth flying into Finland, seeing the Oodi and flying out again.

Finnish Education

The story of how education became the cause célèbre here in the land of concrete and lakes is that about a hundred years ago Finland was incredibly poor from being raped and looted by Russia. The younger generation were moving away to Canada and the US so the country was abandoned as a home for the elderly. Some bright spark came up with the idea that since Finland had nothing concrete to offer (I beg to differ), they would create the best educational system in the world, and they did and the world's people came to find out how it's done.

Now tourists no longer talk about the food (herring – no comment), clothes (sacks and rubber clogs) or accommodation (Soviet and smells like your grandmother); the schools are the most interesting aspect of life. Where America's motto must be 'more is more', Finland's motto is 'less is more'. They start school age seven, arrive at 9 a.m. and leave at 2 p.m. (civilized or what?) with little or no homework, because, guess what, you learn what you need to at school from your teacher and fellow students, not from Mommy or Daddy or tutors. Also, studies have shown that whether you start a kid at five or seven doesn't have any effect on his reading; as a matter of fact, if they start too early, they may resist reading later on.

The reason taxes are high in Finland (which no one I met seemed to mind) is to ensure everyone gets a high-quality education. I mean everyone. I had a Congolese taxi driver who said as soon as he immigrated to Finland, rather than extradite him, they made him go straight to school and paid him for it. This means it isn't a country full of stupid people (see my country). Finland ranked first in the 2016 World Economic Forum human capital index, which was judged on how effective a country was at helping all its citizens fulfil their potential as workers and people.

6 July 2019

I went to the home of Petter Elo, teacher at Hiidenkivi comprehensive school, to find out what's so special about education here. Also, I wanted to see how he lives (he's rich). Teachers are extremely well paid; it's considered a prestigious job and they rank primary school teachers as top of the professions people look for in an ideal partner. His home is in a forest (again) – very Hamsteady-looking.

It's decorated in that Finnish minimalist style: an ice rink of oak floor, enclosed by walls of windows looking out at evergreens. It's decorated with a futuristic chair in the far distance. They don't like clutter so one chair is enough and a tiny table with nothing on it. This chair is so futuristic, you don't know whether to stand, straddle or have sex with it.

He told me the emphasis of the country was to raise good human beings and that the idea is to create a society where you feel free to question things. If it's narrow-minded it's not democratic. Question everything, ask stupid questions. Life is not about knowing the right answers. (Socrates would have agreed.)

Later on, I met the Minister for Education at the hamburger bar of his choice. It was like sitting with a celebrity, people seemed to want to hug him and endlessly came up, thanking him for the work he's doing. He'd got ketchup down his front but didn't seem to care; a total human, not a hint of politician about him. He explained that their mission at schools isn't to create Nobel Prize winners or big industrialists, they want everyone to feel that they count and to make each kid (and adult) feel safe and equal (women have equality with men in all professions) and be part of the community.

Petter explained that the kids in Finland learn to question their desires, asking themselves, 'Do I really need this? Do I really need to buy a new one? Will this make me happier?' They start teaching this to their kids when they're around three years old, at the age that most Western kids learn the 'I want, I want' mantra of consumerism. He told me that at the school he taught at, they still have to follow a curriculum but, more important, they also learn how to think. They may not be able to keep up with a Chinese kid in maths but at skills like complex problem solving or critical thinking, they would leave them in the dust. No cookie-cutter kids found here.

7 July 2019

I need to mention what happened today. It's not about education but I think it's equally important. Max and I had stayed in an Airbnb and at this point Max had left me, so the man who owned the flat asked if I wanted to go riding at his stables. He told me his wife was a showjumper. I do not know why this came out of my mouth, but I said, 'So am I.' It turns out I'm not a showjumper, but I didn't know that at that point. Anyway, he drove me out of town to his other home where there were stables for about twenty horses. Everyone in this country is rich, by the way, but they are kind of humble with it.

So I began by cantering around the ring a few times and then for some strange reason, I do not know why to this day, I decided to take the jump. Now, I've horse-jumped before, years ago, but for some reason I did not obey the jump rules. I leant back and the horse obeyed by stopping sharply, but I didn't. I flew through the air and the noise of my landing was something you should never have to hear in your life, but every bone was involved. Being a Finn, he didn't show much emotion, just said, 'Everyone has bad days.' So unAmerican – he didn't worry about a lawsuit even when I couldn't walk. He moved me like a broken puppet and shoved codeine in me before I started screaming. Somehow he drove me back to the flat, brought me food and a girdle.

Later, after he'd left me at his flat, I had to navigate my way to the bathroom on my knees in the dark. I couldn't reach the light switch and ended up falling down some stairs, which is when my back said, 'Okay, I'm broken now, you've gone too far, I give up.' I decided to leave Finland earlier than I was booked to but not before I went to visit the school I'd arranged to visit. Yes, even though I was going to be disabled for the rest of my life, that's how committed I was to writing this book (though I was on a lot of codeine so maybe I was out of my mind; certainly I was in bliss).

8 July 2019

In the morning I called an Uber driver and said I'd pay him extra if he came upstairs. When he entered the flat, I asked him to pack my suitcase, giving him directions on how to fold the undies. Then I made him carry me and the luggage down the stairs. Only in Finland would this not be considered weird. So he lugged me into the taxi to take me to Kilonpuisto school and the students I was visiting, dragged me out at the other end like an old sack and placed me on floor cushions.

From the floor, I met Susanna Ahvalo, an innovator in teaching emotional skills and self-awareness. She let me lie there for the day.

She explained that she stays with the same class, same students, for six years so they're like family. By law, the classes are all mixed ability. There are no rows of desks in the school rooms. (Rows always remind me of cattle in an abattoir.) Here, the kids sit in a circle and within that circle is another circle. Susanna watches from a distance, doesn't interfere, just steps in to guide once in a while.

The learning comes from the power of the group, they do all their work as a team and this is drilled into them, so if one kid is slower, it behoves the group to help them. She explained to me that the inner circle discusses a topic like what to do about the climate crisis (these kids are ten). They were encouraged to think way out of the box, so the crazier the idea, the better. When the inner group finished, after a set time, they turned to the person behind them in the outer circle and had a discussion. The outer circle fed back their observations on how well the first group listened, whether they made good eye contact and whether they dominated or let others speak. (Children learn better from peers than from teachers. Why didn't we ever think of that?)

The class then brought in their projects. Weeks earlier, they decided it would be Vikings. Each kid could choose which area about the Vikings excited them most; even if you wanted to learn how to pillage that would be fine. In the previous weeks they were sent out like little detectives to find their own way of expressing the life of Vikings. They could shoot a video, write a script, sew the outfits, cook, sing, dance, paint, sculpt. And the kid with the wildest ideas doesn't get bullied like they might anywhere else, because in this school eccentrics rule. Rather than regurgitating some historical information, they are finding their own way to get a taste of what life might have been like back then, even if it's not accurate. (Who knows what's accurate anyway? History isn't accurate, it's a story.) There is no test on Vikings, they all pass and they evaluate how they think they did by giving themselves grades.

When the kids get older, Susanna explained, they begin to introduce a programme that includes being tested for university, but before that creativity is everything. At this young age, they have no fear and don't think of the future, so why scare them about what's coming – let them have fun while they still can.

I was carried into another class, where they'd set up a business village. Each kid had picked an occupation: a grocery store owner, a teacher, a plumber, a clothes manufacturer, an entrepreneur, a video-game maker. Then they research by interviewing people who have the relevant job. At the follow-up presentation, the kids have to explain how they would run their business and how much they would pay themselves and their employees in order to be fair. I was told that what they're learning is not about financial profit but personal profit; how would they use business to have a nice life? Can you imagine suggesting this technique at Harvard Business School? You'd be shot out of the window by a cannon.

They have recesses between every class. Susanna said that after a class their brains are clouded from learning and they need to play throughout the day to recharge their minds.

The most impressive class was watching Susanna teach them how to deal with their emotions, using fairy tales as mindfulness exercises. To begin, she had them lie on the floor and instructed them to put a toy on their stomachs, as in the .b course, watching how their breath affected the movements. They were told to be aware when the toy was jumpy and when it slowed down and barely moved. They raised their hands when they felt the toy calming down. Then she told them the story of 'The Little Mermaid'. She told me this is the way she teaches them how to deal with disappointment. She asks them how the mermaid might feel when the prince leaves her for the princess. They all pitch in – 'anger', 'sadness', 'loneliness'. Susanna asks what those words feel like – 'sweating', 'shaking', 'stabbing'. She hands them all paper with an outline of a body on it and asks them to draw where in the body they feel those sensations; giving them colour, shape, texture. Then she asks what the thoughts are that go with the feelings – 'I hate him', 'I want to tell my mother', 'I want to disappear' – followed by what actions those thoughts and feelings would motivate them to do.

One girl said, 'I would kill him.' (That would be my answer too.) At the end, they discussed if those actions would make the feelings and thoughts go away or would they just keep the cycle pinballing of thoughts, feelings, emotions, actions? Susanna asked them to come up with a solution for the Little Mermaid to help her deal with her situation that would help ease her feeling of disappointment.

These kids are learning how to stand back and observe their feelings and thoughts, and not lash out because of them. They're learning, in spite of the discomfort and pain, not to react but to reflect and come up with clear-minded solutions. One of the kids came up with a great strategy, which was to tell herself it was a lucky break that she didn't marry the prince because if she had, she'd have had to give up her tail and no longer be a mermaid, which would be such a bummer. Then, they made a new chart of their thoughts and emotions in the light of the new solution; much more peaceful. (My favourite girl stuck to her guns with, 'I would still murder him.') Susanna said that that exercise also works a treat with 'The Ugly Duckling', where the kids have to come up with coping mechanisms for the duck; she said it's great for problems with low self-esteem. Who has low self-esteem in Finland? No one. First of all, they all look like blond gods and then it's the happiest country in the world.

After that point, I don't know what happened, but when I woke up, my toy was still on my stomach and I could tell I had been snoring. They gently carried me out to a taxi where I was whisked to the airport. What I mainly learnt from all this superior Finnish style of education was that I will never ride a horse ever again.

4

Technology

When it comes to the future, there are so many things to fear (global warming, inequality, plastic, China and the man who runs America who I still won't name), and obviously these items weren't enough to quench our insatiable hunger for things that scare the pants off of us, so now, Ladies and Gentlemen, let me introduce you to . . . (drum roll) THE FUTURE OF TECHNOLOGY!!

I'm talking about our fear of what's in store for us, like that pretty soon robots are going to suck out our data, splat it on to a USB stick and shove it into a tin can version of ourselves. One of the reasons robots may become more popular than us is because they don't complain, they work 24/7, don't let emotions get in their way, don't die and never get pregnant. They can recognize patterns and calculate possibilities far better than us, without emotions getting in the way. We make mistakes because we rely on a brain that's partially left over from the Stone Age. Fear, frustration or anger trigger those primitive reactions and all rational thinking hits the dust.

By the way, this anxiety about change isn't a new thing. Throughout history, every time we created a new tool, people thought it was the end of the world. Starting with Socrates, whining on, saying that writing would kill our capacity to remember anything and distance us from the truth. He wasn't that smart, contrary to popular belief, he just had a good agent (Plato wrote his lines).

When books came along, people thought we wouldn't be able to speak any more. When we developed the bicycle, train, car, plane, we all worried that it would be the end of walking. Some people thought the radio, TV and phone marked the end of face-to-face contact.

The History of Our Upgrades

My belief is that it was inevitable we would create this technology because our survival depended on us developing the know-how to make the tools we needed.

Throughout our history we've always evolved (genetically, biologically, neurologically, emotionally, psychologically and physically) to keep up with an ever-changing and over-challenging environment. Upgrading is in our DNA.

Millions of years ago, predators grew too big for us to strangle with our hands, so our brains developed an area that gave us the capability to defend ourselves. I don't know which came first, brain growth or tool-making skills or if they were weirdly synchronized. We needed to get meat and, let's not kid ourselves, punching something fifty times bigger than us with pointy teeth didn't really cut it, so almost overnight we began to whittle spears. Because lions got fangs, bulls got horns, we got nothin' to defend ourselves with. At some point we couldn't digest raw meat and it was too tough to swallow so, with absolutely no instruction manual, we made fire.

The next big human upgrade happened when it became apparent that our communication methods, which were primarily grunts, couldn't be understood by neighbouring tribes. Nit-picking wasn't enough to show you cared so we invented language and from then on we never shut up. You couldn't hear yourself think there was so much yabbering. At the same time, regions in our brain developed which allowed sounds to become words and words sentences. With language we could gossip (it was possible with hand signals but too public) and for a while everything was dandy, but because we had now migrated every which way across the globe, we couldn't keep up with the latest scandals. So *voilà*: the written word. Not easy because at the start, writing was in tablet form and who knew how to chisel? Not many. And who could lift that thing? Even Moses put his back out trying. Luckily, someone invented papyrus in Egypt which spread like wildfire, no name because he forgot to sign his first work. By the way, a bit later someone else thought of using a feather for a pen and from then on no turkey was safe. It really caught on; Shakespeare, Milton and Jackie Collins all managed to create the greatest literature the world has ever known with a mere plume and no 'delete' button. Have you seen the Bible? Who the hell managed all those words without one mistake? But as you all know, this great literature wasn't spreading fast enough, because how many times could you expect Shakespeare to copy the same play over and over again to make it on to the bestseller list, without his hand getting paralysed? So . . . enter the printing press. As luck would have it, in 1455, Johannes Gutenberg invented printing by movable type.

My point is we are first suspicious of new gadgets and then we love them.

My Story

I remember how happy I was when mobiles first appeared; hands free at last, free at last. You could talk anywhere, any time. We no longer had to run like slaves to pick up the phone anchored to a kitchen wall or perched on a side table. And best of all, mobiles have liberated us from needing to use payphones (telephone boxes to you). In the days I first got here to the UK (on the *Mayflower*'s return journey) they were on every street corner; red, coffin-sized and cracked windowed with phones that never worked. You had to shove a steady flow of coins into the slots like you were playing Vegas on a losing streak. I guess it didn't matter that you never connected to anyone because the phone booths were mainly used for people to pee and vomit in on Saturday night. Now they're in museums like great works of art. They were hellholes!

The Bad News

I know I said this book will try to show the good news in the future but I don't want to appear naive, so I'm going to give you some bad news because someone else will tell you and it might as well be me. In the future, I don't know exactly when – I'm not a psychic like everyone else seems to be – but in the next few decades it's estimated that nearly 47 per cent of jobs, the equivalent of about 37.7 million people, may become redundant because of a robotic workforce. Start drinking the titanium.

But don't worry . . . this isn't the first time our livelihoods have been threatened. Just so you're not shaking in your boots at this point, let me mention that on the eve of the

1900s over 40 per cent of the workforce was employed in agriculture. Now it is less than 2 per cent.

Jobs That will be Replaced by Robots

Accountants They have a 95 per cent chance of losing their jobs to automation in the future. I never loved accountants anyway – they charge too much and never give you good news.

Drivers Fleets of autonomous vehicles will replace human taxi drivers, truck drivers and other transportation jobs. Don't get cocky, you'll be made redundant too by driverless cars.

Chefs Chef Watson is a robot who can generate new recipes from scratch, and Miso Robotics' burger-making Flippy can prepare meals and serve them up much quicker than humans. Then a table delivery drone can serve it to the customer. (Bye-bye, waitresses.)

Financial analysts Computers can spot patterns and make trades faster than humans. These guys predict 30 per cent of the banking sector jobs will be lost to AI within the next decade. Does that make me sad? No, I'd rather be ripped off by a machine than a banker.

Manual labour An automated bricklayer can lay up to 1,200 bricks a day, compared to the 300–500 a human can.

Farmers Cows can now mosey up to a robot when they want to be milked rather than you having to herd them and then piss them off. The robot is, hopefully, gentle on the udders.

Receptionists and phone operators A robot can just as easily say, 'I'll put you on hold.' Or 'Have a nice day.'

Pilots US Military are using autonomous drones that conduct surveillance and attacks without the assistance of humans. Do you feel safer now?

Safe Jobs That Can't Be Replaced

Recreational therapists
Mental health and substance abuse social workers
Occupational therapists
Healthcare social workers
Masseurs

If I were you, I'd start studying to be a therapist now because clearly we're going to need lots of them. I'm sure the reaction to redundancy is full-tilt horror. I'm not saying it isn't, we need to survive, but running scared won't solve the problem. Our fear of mass unemployment isn't new either – in 1930 the economist Maynard Keynes predicted that by 2030 most people's jobs would be replaced by technology and all we would have to do would be to find wonderful and fulfilling things to do with our leisure time. Flower-pressing, rock-collecting, mushroom-picking, etc. But what he didn't predict was our insatiable addiction to wanting more stuff and the fact that in the last fifty years people's jobs have become their identity. 'How ya doin'?' has been replaced by 'What do you do?' Most people don't really seem to care how you are but they do want to know how much money you make. Babies and elderly people are probably the only ones not asked, 'And what do you do?' Though when my daughter, Marina, was five and told me she had a boyfriend, I asked, 'What does he do for a living?' See? I'm part of the problem. I'm so ashamed.

More About Robots

Anyway, back to robots . . . We are now entering the Second Machine Age. (The first one was when Scottish inventor James Watt came up with the steam engine. In those days we were using tech to save our muscles; now we use it to replace brain work.) New generations of robots are taking over. Ray Kurzweil (more on him shortly) says that by 2029 computers will be as intelligent as people. By 2045 they may be a billion times smarter than all human brains put together. You can kick and scream all you want about this technological revolution, but it was inevitable just like that spear that had to be whittled. And what's more extraordinary is that along with these inventions, we've evolved specific parts of our brains simultaneously that not only help us make the appropriate tools but also learn how to use them. Just think, our kids are already genetically modified with faster reaction times to keep up with high-speed computers. Their motor cortex is thicker in the area of the brain that's associated with the fingers, which is why they are so adept. Let me explain on the sciencey level because it's my happy place. There's a region in your brain (somatosensory cortex) with a map of all your body parts on it. The bigger the area in the brain, the more proficient you are when using the corresponding part of your body. Dancers have more real estate on the feet area. Porno stars have bigger terrain representing their genitalia (you probably can tell how well someone is hung just by checking on a brain scanner). Violinists, Chinese children who sew zippers into your shorts and kids who play a lot of video games all have a huge plot of property in Finger-ville. My generation will never have the dexterity of a four-year-old but don't worry because we'll have our revenge; our kids will be panicking like we did when their children come home with chip implants.

So our fear of technology is nothing new. When I was growing up, people reported sightings of flying saucers, and they thought aliens were going to hoover them into the mothership and make them slaves. (They still believe this in certain parts of Tennessee.) What we actually worry about is that robots are going to turn evil and annihilate our species and there is talk of people 'getting uploaded', which is the conversion of the human mind into software. I've read about something coming our way in the future called the 'Omega Point'. (I'll have to quote because you'll think I'm making it up.) 'It is a projection whereby intelligent life takes over all matter in the universe, leading to a cosmological singularity which will allow future societies to resurrect the dead.' Leaf through a book called, *The Singularity is Near* by Ray Kurzweil. (Yes, it's Ray again but now he's on acid.) The book is so thick and complex that unless you're a robot you won't understand a word. You have to hack through a jungle of quantum physics, incomprehensible equations and mathematical scribble. At the heart of a billion words, I think he's trying to say that in the year 2024 at 4.00 a.m. or thereabouts, our consciousness will be sent to the Cloud and we will all become cyborgs. Human Body Version 3.0. Post-singularity there will be no distinction between human and machine or between physical and virtual reality. Ray knows all this because he is Google's chief futurist and so he must be telling the truth.

A new group of people are calling themselves trans-humanists, who define themselves as, 'A liberation movement, advocating nothing less than a total emancipation from biology itself.' The final frontier between the convergence of technology and flesh.

About a decade and a half ago, we worshiped those Uber-geeks of Silicon Valley, those titans of technology. Now we paint them with the same brush as we do Genghis Khan, Vlad the Impaler and our own loonie in the White House: The Trumpster.

Let's remember, tech wasn't forced on us. We lined up around the block for the latest iPhone, we feasted on more and more bytes until they became gigabytes which then became zillionabytes and maybe now a jillion, jillion bytes, squared. What's so typical of human nature is that we've turned on the very people who invented these digital miracles. Now, when we're not using our fingers to push keys, we're using them to point at Silicon Valley, blaming them for destroying our minds and, even more, our children's minds. May I make a small point here? If I'm not mistaken, we still have the power to literally pull the plug or just simply switch our machine or phone to 'off'. The choice is still ours.

Where It Might Have Gone Wrong

Despite the bad press they get, I know that Facebook, Google and Amazon started off as meaning well; to give us connection with everyone, anywhere, and download us instantaneous information about everything that exists. With a simple click on the 'buy what's in the basket now' icon, you can have it all; almost anything on earth delivered straight into your mouth or really any orifice of your choice. The net originally gave us peer-to-peer connections and free expression and turned us back into a collective, just like the old days when we sat around the fire, sharing gossip. I read that Zuckerberg created Facebook to link all his fellow students at Harvard so they could exchange ideas and gossip. Just as our ancient ancestors created language when they needed to dish the dirt, this guy built something that could send gossip to a billion people at once. To be exact, in

2019 he had 2.4 billion users worldwide, adding 500,000 new users every day. Six new profiles every second, that's a lot of gossip.

I'll bet Instagram's Mike Krieger just wanted to share photos of nice vistas to make his friends feel happy. He didn't think someday Instagram would be used by some asshole posing on a yacht framed by babes' backsides. Even the guys who started Snapchat probably just wanted to send out photos of their genitals and, knowing that the image would disappear after thirty seconds, didn't mean any harm. They all just wanted to spread a little goodness in the world, a little joy.

In 2009 Justin Rosenstein and Leah Pearlman were part of a small team at Facebook that designed the 'like' button, a little blue-and-white thumbs-up designed to give you a hit of confidence with a pinch of positivity. They had no idea that someday people would judge their own worth on whether a thumb went up or down nor that if they received too many thumbs-down it would seriously damage their health. (There should be a warning sign next to the down thumbs, like the ones they show on the cigarette packets of bleeding gums and people's tarred organs.) I read in an article that Leah now makes Buddhist comics and says she regrets having ever unleashed that thumb on the world.

I'm sure the creators of tech didn't imagine that the same net that connected us would now be isolating us from each other. But once these innocent little apps and icons took over the world, the creators sold out and turned their inventions into big business. I guess if you're twenty and are sitting in your garage watching your bank balance go from zilch to millions, it is enough to make you crazy. Very few people ever say, 'I have enough money, let's stop here.' Who knows when Zuckerberg got greedy. I guess it began when he thought he needed a bigger sofa and some new cushions; once he realized he could manipulate the user and also sell private information to advertisers, he knew he'd hit gold.

The Evil of Ads

Enter the advertisers and data hackers. As soon as you have advertising, manipulation steps into the picture to convince you (the sucker) to buy something you don't need. When an advertiser tells us, 'Oh come on, everyone wants sneakers that cost £700,' I say to them, 'You are the devil.'

Ad men (see *Mad Men*) in the 1950s just about got away with ads on television because you were aware of them and had a choice: to stay and watch or leave the room to raid the fridge. Now advertisers know how to sell you things no matter what room you're in.

What began as an innocent ad has now morphed into continuous behaviour modification on a mass level. In my humble opinion, people online are under surveillance through their devices receiving calculated zaps of influence that gradually change who they are. If this is true, we're as good as lab rats who, as we all know, will even learn to pole dance if they get electrically zapped enough. We aren't aware of any of this, but even if the on-screen pop-up suggestions are innocent now (telling us what clothes to buy, based on our personal data), maybe in the future they will influence our decisions on who we marry, what religion to follow and who to vote for. Taking away our need to make decisions removes our meaning and free will. Can you imagine, Hamlet says, 'To be or not to be?' and his computer squawks out the answer (based on what colour jerkin he's wearing and if he's seen a ghost or not).

Tickling Our Addiction Buttons

Our phones and computers make us junkies, offering us a fix that never fixes and leaving us in a state of craving; we can never quite scratch this insatiable itch and on our brains there's a tattoo that reads, 'It's never enough.'

Obviously certain drugs are habit forming, but today's addictions to texting, sexting and instagramming, etc., though these things are not addictive in themselves, still stimulate the dopamine you manufacture in your brain to make you want to shoot up Twitter or snort Snapchat.

And you don't need physical rewards, even an image can get you hooked as the advertisers cleverly understand. A smartphone game like *Candy Crush* uses shiny images of candy instead of real candy to get you craving; video games, like gambling machines, use images of coins or treasure chests and any sign of a positive emoji to reinforce your hunger. We look for solace in a square or rectangular piece of metal for a few measly hits of happiness. That's why some people check their phone 1,467 times a day.

Social status and feedback from others online has there-fore become a primal need; we've become slaves to a smiley face. I'm not being smug, I'm as befuddled as you are as to where to draw the line. I badly need the laptop which I'm typing on at this very moment to write this book. How else would I do that? With a plume and a pigeon to deliver it to your door? Forget it. I can't write without this computer, but what makes me insane is that while I'm typing this very word, every cell in my body wants to check my in-box. The computer isn't forcing me or flashing, 'Check the emails,' it's habit and my fear of being forgotten, and the more I find in my in-box, the more loved I feel, even if it's spam.

Back to Zuckerberg and his need for a bigger sofa . . .

Besides selling your private thoughts, he brought in mathematicians and engineers to create algorithms. The definition, for those of you like me who have no idea what an algorithm is: 'a set of mathematical instructions or rules that, given to a computer, will calculate an answer to a problem.' These algorithms can create a portfolio of who you are by detecting patterns for figuring out your heart's desires and then you can be monetized by 'growth hackers', who in the end will know you better than your best bestie. Then 'data hackers' harvest that information, put it in farms (don't imagine cow stalls, imagine thousands of computers humming day and night) and sell it to opinion makers (see Cambridge Analytica) who pay a high price for your personal information. They can then modify which images to flash on to your screen, based on your desires, to make you vote how they want you to or to reach for your credit card.

This business model guarantees that persuasion will always be the default goal of every design. Every pixel on every screen has been tuned to influence users' actions and create addictions. And here's the rub: when we're caught in online addiction, it lowers our quality of life, lowers our IQ and lowers our ability to focus. As I said, we little humans can't win against these weapons of mass distraction. I don't want to add to your fear, but I must. I read in a PC mag that on average in the UK people spend nearly 6 hours per day on media and 3.9 of that is on smartphones, checking them every 12 minutes. That means we spend a quarter of our waking lives on a mobile device. (I don't know how they gather this data. Does someone run from house to house with a stopwatch?) There's a word for our addiction: 'nomophobia' – fear of being without a phone.

It is your choice if you want to sell a kidney or some other vital organ, but your attention is being stolen without your permission. Attention will be the bitcoin of the blockchain of our currency in the future. Netflix too is an expert on making us addicts. I'm up all night, helplessly hitting the 'next episode' icon, and when a series ends, I have actual cold turkey withdrawal; Netflix is in our bloodstream now. When you socialize no one talks about anything except what series they're hooked on. It's like drug addicts exchanging tips on best methods for shooting up.

A Fantasy

Here's a crazy idea for the future or, heck, even right now. Let's imagine that Zuckerberg (pretend he has enough sofas) suddenly says:

'Okay, Facebook is not going to be a listed business any more. We said we wanted to create this thing to connect people, but we're actually making the world worse, so we're not gonna allow people to advertise or allow any third party to have any influence on you. We're gonna turn it into a non-profit; we're gonna give it to each country; it'll be nationalized.'

We can all dream.

So Finally Some Green Shoots: When Tech is Good, It's Very, Very Good

On the plus side, technology is what's saving lives and making education, knowledge, communication and connection accessible to everyone on earth. I have watched TED Talks and scoured reports on new inventions (so you don't have to) and here's what's coming down the line to make you feel better about the tech future.

In Medicine

In the near future, tattoos on your skin will transmit your biological condition directly to your doctor who can shoot you back medication wirelessly without you even being awake. It seems sci-fi at the moment but the technology to do this is already in development. I can only imagine what this will look like. Imagine being in serious trouble and an ambulance is remotely alerted to collect you or, in my worst-case scenario, a hearse shows up at your door. But seriously, scientists will be able to tweak your genes and deliver the right medication straight to you. Grains of sand-sized capsules will be able to roam your insides through the bloodstream, hunting for foreign objects that don't belong there, and then shoot them down like an internal video game.

They can already analyse DNA in cancer cells and, using special algorithms, a computer can amalgamate your data and mix you a personalized bespoke medication, the drone can deliver it to your door (and maybe wax your legs or shoot you some Botox while it's there). When you're not using your 3D printer to make household appliances and car parts, you can make yourself a bespoke kidney, just in case, so you've got a spare.

The blind will soon be able to throw away the stick and dog (sorry, dogs, you're out of a job too), and have a bionic eye made from a 3D printer in an hour. Eye lenses packed with biosensors will be engineered to pick up early detection of diabetes by measuring blood sugar in tears. If you happen to have a missing limb, they will make you a new improved one that guarantees you a place in the Paralympics. While you're sleeping, electrodes in your pillowcase and sheets will collect information by monitoring brainwaves. Toothbrushes will be able to give you instant results by interpreting your saliva. Smart refrigerators will monitor food and record nutritional information. A smart bra will be able to detect breast cancer. A selfie from a smartphone app will be able to diagnose pancreatic cancer by analysing the whites of your eyes. Microsurgery is already being done by robotic arms that are more accurate than any human capability and they don't shake. If you can imagine it, they've invented it.

And on the brain front: the use of implanted electrodes to deliver electric pulses known as deep brain stimulation, which is already having positive results with Parkinson's, OCD and other mental illnesses such as depression. (Whoever has access to one of those electrodes: I'll pay, please, I'm begging.) Also, smartphones will be able to detect depression or other mental illnesses and notify your doctor.

To me, this next one is a jaw-dropper of medical invention: Manu Prakash, physicist and inventor, makes microscopes out of paper. Most people in the world don't have access to a lab with microscopes to test samples for diseases. Thanks to Manu, you get a piece of cardboard, embedded with every component in a microscope, and fold it, like making a paper doll (the instructions are colour coded so you don't even need to read). This disposable origami-looking thing can identify tiny life forms that cause infectious diseases, such as malaria, tuberculosis, HIV/AIDS, pneumonia, hepatitis B and C, and now the latest on the block, coronavirus.

If this is all on the horizon, I say bring in the robots, AI and apps.

Sustainable Innovations for Consumers and for the Planet

Daniel Goleman, author of *Ecological Intelligence*, talks about apps in the near future which will display data, as a simple readout, to give us the hidden impacts of what we buy, sell or make on the health of the environment. The name and age of the person who sewed the zipper into your pants, how many pollutants are actually in your new dog-hair blower or whether the chicken you're eating was a criminal. When we know all this, then and only then will the power shift from those who sell to those who buy.

An emerging idea is to put stickers on products with a code, which if you punch it into your computer will give you direct access to both the farmer and the manufacturer who grew or produced it. And once we CAN find out who are the wrongdoers, we just tweet the bad guys to death with a ThisSucksandThisRules hashtag. This is 'radical transparency' at its best. The millennials are wired to each other unlike any other generation, that's why a photo of a cat getting married can be seen by millions before the bride even gets to the end of the aisle.

Suzanne Lee does a great TEDTalk on biofabrication which she says is the 'fourth industrial revolution'. She started her business by designing what she calls bio-couture; crossing fashion with biology. Instead of following the usual processing of plants, animals and oil to make consumer products, she grows materials using living organisms like bacteria, fungi, yeast and algae. So instead of having to grow cotton in fields, you grow microbes, over several months, to make a similar material. Suzanne then cuts out the pattern in this sheath of microbes for making shoes, bags and clothes. (I'm wondering, when you get tired of an outfit, can you just eat it?) You don't need to ship or fly these materials all over the world, you grow them in a lab, making zero waste.

Mycelium is a kind of fungi which is multi-cellular and feeds off sugars and starches to grow. This can be rapid – after two weeks' growth you can have a sheet (18' × 12' × 2') that can then be manipulated into building anything you can imagine. If you take a 3D mould and fill it with waste products like corn stalks, add water and wait a few days for the mycelia to grow, you're producing living organisms that can be turned into phones, buildings, furniture, flooring, etc. 'Grow your own home' would be my suggestion for a slogan. Fungi is a material that can grow with no chemicals added, it's water absorbent, fire resistant and can be composted in your back garden. Instead of using cement to make bricks for building houses, causing 8 per cent of global CO_2 emissions (more than planes and ships each year), you can grow bio-bricks which are three times stronger than a concrete block and store carbon. If we can replace the 1.2 trillion fired bricks made each year with their bio-brick brothers, it reduces CO_2 emissions by 800 million tonnes every year.

We know the hazards of using plastic bags and yet almost everything we buy is already gift-wrapped in them. In the US alone, 8 billion are used each year, they're blowing in the breeze from Santiago to Siberia. It's like cigarettes, we all knew the warnings but kept on lighting up. And then one day, they were gone (except in France) and it suddenly wasn't cool to smoke like it was in high school, when the most popular kids puffed in the toilets. There are already substitutes for plastic, but do we hear about them? No, we do not, unless we go trolling through websites.

Seaweed

In 2018, seaweed, which can grow 3 metres a day, has emerged as another alternative to oil-based plastic. As well as being abundant – just 0.03 per cent of the brown seaweed in the world could replace all of the polyethylene terephthalate (PET) plastic bottles we get through every year – it can solve what is known as shelf-life gap, the difference between the biodegradability of a container and whatever is in it. For example, instead of using the demon plastic water bottle, how about Edible Blobs (they are really called that) filled with water? They look like rubbery bubbles and are made from this seaweed extract. You're thirsty? You just pop one in your mouth, it's that easy. And you can probably throw them at people to give yourself a laugh.

This begs the question, why aren't these alternatives to plastic seen on every shop shelf? Why don't they pop up on your computer screen, instead of portable Zimmer frames? Each new sustainable invention should be in the headlines of every newspaper, every day of the week, around the world, not what's killing us next. I don't want to write about conspiracy theories but I can't help wondering whether big conglomerates are giving hush money or, dare I say, bribing politicians (who could probably reroute the eco disaster) to turn a blind eye and keep the 'Good Ol' Boys' swimmin' in oil. I don't want to write about it because I don't want to be bumped off.

Some World Changers

- Already on the market are plastic bags that dissolve in water, made from cassava, a starch that is shown to be harmless for animal consumption; so once dissolved, you can drink them if you're in the mood.
- Tech Insider reported that a company called Liter of Light in the Philippines have created street lights made from used plastic bottles filled with bleach and water then fixed to rooftops; or, if fitted with a micro-solar panel inside, they can light a house. They already light 850,000 homes

around the world and they aim to provide for a million soon.

- Desalination, where saltwater is made drinkable, is now being made more effective by a giant sieve made out of graphene. Since 2004 a Manchester-led team have developed this technology to make a membrane with tiny (less than a nanometre) holes to filter out the sodium chloride, only letting the water molecules through.

- To compensate for the decreasing population of bees, a drone can help plants to pollinate. In Japan, Eijiro Miyako and his colleagues have used the principle of cross-pollination in bees to make a drone that transports pollen between flowers. He started off trying this with lilies but is now working on a variation to pollinate crops.

- The Seabin Project in Sydney collects garbage from the sea by using a pump to create a flow of water that sucks rubbish inside the bin like a hoover. There's a sieve-like bag inside the Seabin that's lifted out for emptying, allowing water to flow back into the sea.

- Edible spoons taste like crackers made from millet, rice and wheat. If you throw them in the ocean, fish like them too. And if they could say 'Bon appétit' they would.

- Saltwater Brewery has created edible packaging to save sea life. The six-pack rings are made of barley and wheat which again sea creatures can eat till the cows come home.

- Waterlily is a turbine or power generator you can hold in your hand to harvest energy, off-grid, from a river and charge any device. The faster the water flows the more power you can generate and you can get electricity night and day. Great for hikers/campers/those who live beside rivers.

- SpinCycle is a small machine filled with a little water which you hook on to the back of your bike. As you pedal, the machine spins, washing your clothes as you ride. This is aimed at people in developing countries and those of us on the go, who don't have time to do our laundry.

- At MIT media lab they invented a device that captures air pollution and then turns it into ink. Known as Air-Ink, it collects carbon soot from cars' exhaust and then it's processed into a high-quality black ink. The particulate matter (soot to you and me) that belches out of cars, chimneys, etc., is captured and cleaned of carcinogens and heavy metals, and then, *voilà*, you are left with black ink.

- The Ocean Cleanup, an organization from the Netherlands, has designed a giant ocean boom to scoop up debris. The flexible pipe moves with the waves and has floating anchors, and when the plastic waste is all gathered into a central island, a boat comes to remove it. At the time of writing, this is in its infancy as they have had glitches to sort out, but they hope to launch a total of sixty such systems by 2021.

Quantum Computers

Nothing but nothing competes with this tech of all techs that's going to change the future forever: quantum computing. (I have to make it simple because I don't really understand it and failed at maths. But I do know Hartmut Neven, personally, who heads the Google quantum department and made one of the first quantum computers. We met at Burning Man which qualifies me as an expert now.)

He explained that the first actual quantum computer is being stored at NASA where it's kept cold, as in ten 'millikelvin' (Hartmut knows what that is), to run the quantum processors, and it can do in 220 seconds what the world's biggest supercomputer called Summit can do in 10,000 years. (It's not a typo.)

The computers we use now reflect how our brains solve problems, imitating our neural relay system; just as our 86 billion neurons pass information via electrical currents, so too do they communicate through electrical impulses, each zapping the next. That's why you can type in anything and up pops whatever you desire. Everything from how to do heart surgery on a racoon to finding a pizzeria in Tonga.

Quantum computing doesn't emulate the processes in our brains, it mimics nature and nature knows everything. A tree knows how to turn carbon dioxide into oxygen, it doesn't need to go online. I'm told that in less than a decade, quantum computing will be able to crack the code of how a tree actually does that miraculous trick. Not to mention how these computers will be able to understand nature's algorithms and create a battery that works like the sun without needing cobalt (something that's only available in the Congo) or any other unsustainable material.

While medical research costs trillions, nature (which is free) knows how to make nearly every medicine in the world; you can heal practically anything from what grows on tree bark. If quantum computing can copy nature, we've hit the jackpot.

At this moment, the only way to discover a cure for a disease is to painstakingly, by computer simulation, create endless combinations of molecules, to find the one that binds with the receptor of, say, a specific cancer molecule. After that, some drug company, at great expense, has to develop that molecule which, after a long time, finally goes on to the market. A quantum computer will be able to instantly find what molecule binds with which receptor molecule, therefore finding cures for diseases in a zillionth of the time it takes now.

Evolving Tech to Make Us More Human

Okay, this is my area of interest and the point I'm trying to make is that the innovative technology is coming to relieve our ailing minds, bodies and hopefully the planet, but here's the rub. No matter how great the tech, unless we learn to lower the fear in which we're now saturated, our own stress will kill us by breaking down our immune systems so that we become open house for cancer, diabetes, dementia, strokes and heart attacks, etc.

Also, if we're too fearful, we fall into our egomaniacal mode where we start using tech to gene splice smarter kids or steal stem cells to grow us a better nose. Remember, we'll keep creating chaos if our minds are in chaos.

The only way for us to learn to manage our stress and be able to curb our addictive behaviours is if we change ourselves (not through an app). It can't be done by some quick fix but by training ourselves in self-awareness and self-knowledge, with the same diligence we use when we learn a language.

I think that one of the reasons for our obsession with tech is that it's distracting us from our anger and loneliness and fear of . . . the big one . . . death. For example, if we have insight and learn to calm our minds, we might be less susceptible to being manipulated by advertising. After all, studies have shown that socially fulfilled people need less money, experience less shame, behave less predictably and act more autonomously.

There is already tech for mindfulness; very successful apps such as Headspace and Calm which are used by millions (and worth billions, I'm happy to say) and, no question, these help lasso that mental bucking bronco and calm it down. But eventually you have to take off the training wheels and cold turkey yourself off from the instructions.

As I've said, mindfulness is about being alone with your sometimes unbearable thoughts and, with friendly curiosity, observe them without judgement. The idea is ultimately to see them as mental phenomena, like sounds coming and going without any effort, not taking them personally. You can think of them as like a radio station that randomly plays in the background when you haven't chosen the channel.

It's so easy to get sucked into mass rage, which is the collective weather condition of our culture, making us feel all united in fury, but ultimately being destructive of ourselves and the planet. These mindfulness practices wake us up to the fact that our thoughts are conditioned by a world where our default mindset is materialism and competition. Mindfulness can get to the root of our insecurities that lie behind our fear and loneliness. I said earlier that so far our biology can't keep up with the technology so what we need now are well-meaning coders to build hardware that can help us evolve our own software.

Yuval Noah Harari says, 'For every dollar and every minute we invest in artificial intelligence, we need to invest a dollar and a minute in human consciousness. Otherwise we have upgraded machines which are being controlled by downgraded humans, wreaking havoc on themselves and on the world.' He believes that losing mental autonomy to AI can partly be countered by cultivating mindfulness. In an era where our screens are watching us and stealing our data like digital vampires, he believes we need to be alert to the workings of our minds. Our personal freedom depends on how well we know ourselves because we need to be ahead of the governments or corporations that try to manipulate us. To think clearly is a form of social action.

So, to help us gain inner knowledge, outside of practising mindfulness (which isn't for everyone), I've hand-picked some programmes which are examples of where, I think, tech is working for the good of our mental health.

Joseph Aoun, President of Northeastern University, agrees with me, predicting that we are entering the 'age of humanics', rather than an 'age of robotics', which he defined as: 'An age that integrates our human and technological capacities to meet the global challenges of our time.'

The following apps are not to enhance our cognitive intelligence but our emotional intelligence (which I rate as more important).

Tech to Develop Emotional Intelligence (In My Opinion)

Woebot – Learning to 'Know Thyself'
Alison Darcy at Stanford is the creator of Woebot, the latest technology for Cognitive Behavioural Therapy. She created an interactive robot to help people suffering from depression, anxiety and burnout.

As a solution to CBT, she has created an on-screen bot therapist who gently encourages users to question their 'distorted thinking' by asking the same questions a real CBT therapist would. The bot asks the users to write down their moods, thoughts and emotions in specific situations and then helps them notice if those are old habits or appropriate reactions. Gradually, by becoming aware, you can let go of these unhelpful habits and create more positive ones. I can hear you saying, 'What the fuck? I thought she said robots wouldn't be able to replace therapists?' But in certain situations, with certain therapies, here's why robots aren't such a ridiculous idea.

First of all, Woebot doesn't pretend to be human when it chats to you. It doesn't try to fool you by saying things like, 'I'm going to tell you a little bit about how I like to work with humans.' (It's a no-bullshit bot.) This Woebot is free worldwide and in the first week made more than 50,000 interactions; more people than a human therapist could do in a lifetime. Nowadays, Woebot exchanges between one and two million messages a week with users, especially with young men who often don't seek out therapy and often need it more than most; the highest rate of suicide is among men under forty.

Half the world doesn't have access to basic health care and mental health care is completely inaccessible for many (because either they haven't got money, don't know where to find a good therapist or feel stigmatized).

One in ten people a few years ago had to wait for more than a year to get a mental health assessment and they say by 2030 around two million more people will have a mental health problem, so what's your choice? It's cost-effective, no waiting times and you don't have to leave the house.

Video Games
On average, young kids between the ages of eight and eighteen rack up more than 70 minutes of video gameplay daily. This spike in gameplay happens at the age when kids are most vulnerable to first encounters with depression, anxiety and bullying. So video games generally have a very bad rap these days. Richard Davidson is Professor of Psychology and Psychiatry at the University of Wisconsin. (He was the first doctor to scan the brains of monks who had meditated for more than 10,000 hours and published the phenomenal results.) Now he's doing research on gaming. He says, 'Our long-term aspiration for this work is that video games may be harnessed for good and if the gaming industry and consumers took this message to heart, they could potentially create video games that change the brain in positive ways.'

His games are created for kids who love playing and

parents who'd like to find an alternative that doesn't stoke their addiction, keeping them wired up all night screaming, 'Kill, kill, kill!'

Davidson's team wanted to learn whether there were ways to use video games as a vehicle for positive emotional development during this critical period. They came up with *Crystals of Kaydor*, aimed at developing empathy and emotional intelligence.

A space-exploring robot crashes on a distant planet and in order to gather the pieces of its damaged spaceship and repair it, the player needs to build emotional rapport with the local aliens. The aliens speak a different language but their facial expressions are human-like and are programmed for the players to recognize the six basic emotions: anger, fear, happiness, surprise, disgust and sadness. By watching the avatars' facial expressions and head movements, the player can then respond and, through trial and error, receive feedback through changes in the expression of the avatar. If the avatar feels it's being understood it smiles and continues repairing the spaceship. If it's sad, it doesn't do anything until the child changes his own expression.

As players progress through the game, they go on quests with the avatars and learn how the story impacts on the avatars' emotions.

Davidson and his team researched whether these types of video games could boost kids' empathy, and how that would affect the neural connections in the brain. The team obtained MRI scans and after two weeks of gameplay on *Crystals*, players had stronger connectivity in empathy-related brain networks. (VMPFC, DMPFC and RTP for any neuroscience buffs out there.) So, the more kids play the game, the more they develop those empathy muscles to eventually be able to use as social skills in real life.

Me: A Kid's Diary by Tinybop was developed by a Brooklyn-based app design studio to encourage kids to look inside themselves to explore their emotional states in order to understand themselves better. For example, one of the games on *Me* depicts dark storm clouds and, after tapping on it, *Me* asks how the player feels and to give a colour to that fear. Then an emotional spectrum appears and the app asks questions about the fear, telling them to take a photo of an object that scared them, draw a picture of themselves when they feel fearful and draw a monster that looks like their fear.

Using Virtual Reality for the Good (Empathy Training)

The UN made one of the first virtual reality films to give us the experience of being inside a refugee camp. It is called *Clouds Over Sidra*, where a twelve-year-old Syrian girl takes us on a tour of the camp. We watch her at school, then playing football, and then meet her large family in a one-room tin tent without electricity or hot and cold running anything. She's wonderful and you are charmed. The idea is to create empathy by witnessing a human life, up close and personal. Television just doesn't cut it, a 2D image can't bring it home as well as a 3D twelve-year-old can.

I watched another VR film where I saw Syrian kids running from a fighter jet. I was screaming at them to get down, then when I thought the bombs were dropping, I hunkered under my kitchen table. This is where tech can help to connect humans and move them from self-obsession to world-obsession. Such is the power of VR when used for the good.

Random Acts of Kindness (Connection to Others)

An app called Random App of Kindness (RAKi) helps increase empathetic habits in teens using interactive games designed for smartphones. The goal is that playing with RAKi will help teens develop skills for healthier and more positive social connections. This project is based on epigenetics, the study of how genes can change throughout your life when you change your experiences, so your biology is not your destiny.

This game, like previous ones, teaches empathy by helping players read emotions in others. Various parts of the face come up on the screen and the game asks players to match the eyes, nose and mouth area to an emotion: pain, fear, surprise, joy, etc. It is based on the research of mirror neurons in the brain which create 'motor mimicry', imitating each other's expressions, creating empathy and prosocial behaviours. This also teaches them conflict resolution, a skill the world is badly in need of, while they learn anger management and impulse control to enable them to think clearly even when they want to rip their opponents' throats out.

In the game, the players are faced with an angry man, and rather than flinging their own anger back (which is usually what we do), the players try to get into his shoes.

I think with these apps and games, the creators' hearts and minds are in the right place. We have to start somewhere. The robots can't replace us humans, but if they help stimulate feelings of compassion, it switches on our bonding juice: oxytocin. It's like the foreplay to opening the heart.

No Isolation (Helping with Loneliness)
This is a Norwegian tech company whose stated aim is: 'To reduce involuntary loneliness and social isolation by developing communication tools that help those affected.' They've created a robot to help kids with mental or long-term physical illnesses who are isolated. A robot called AV1, a 'telepresence

bot', takes the place of the child in the classroom, becoming their eyes and ears, communicating with the teacher and classmates. Okay, you may think this is horrifying, using robots as long-distance representatives for kids, but if they can't get out of the house due to mental or physical illness, it's a start. No Isolation has also developed KOMP, which is an easy-to-use smart device to assist the elderly in communicating with their friends and family. No more touch screens or complicated button-pushing, there is a single analogue button to press. It can receive photos and phone calls automatically and is set up in the house like a radio so they can't say they lost it or can't plug it in.

Paro (Pet Alternative)

Paro, developed in Japan by Takanori Shibata, is a robotic fluffy baby seal which recognizes voices, tracks motions and responds with cute little squeaks and whistles. It's a pet alternative for the elderly or anyone who just wants something to cuddle without having to clean up its shit. It wiggles in your arms and is a few degrees warmer than a human. A real pet can scratch or bite whereas Paro only shows love and appreciation when you pet it. My daughter, who is so in love with seals she wants to marry one, almost fainted when she saw Paro. To recharge it, you put a dummy in its mouth just like you would a baby. Okay, I'm getting a little nauseous too . . . but it has amazing results for people with dementia because they may not be able to express affection but they can feel it. The reason it is so popular in Japan may be because of the Shinto belief that spirits can reside in inanimate objects. Need I remind you that we in the West also project love on to objects: a painting, a car, a pair of shoes. So why wouldn't you feel love from and for a toy seal? The good news is it won't ever leave you or die like everything else does.

Technology

*Connect: Human to Human (I invented this app – if you're
an app developer, call me)*
When you log on to this game, you're randomly connected to
another person (a stranger) who can be in any country in the
world. The rules come up on the screen. For the first minute
neither of you speak; you just look at each other, noticing the
eyes, nose, mouth, skin texture, etc. Notice what likes and
dislikes come up for you. The next instruction is for one of
you to speak for three minutes (if it's a foreign language
there's a simultaneous translation), the other just listens. Suggested topics come up on screen which may prompt the
speaker or he/she can just speak spontaneously.

Suggestions:

What did you want to be when you grew up?
Have you accomplished your childhood dreams?
What's your life like now?
What makes you happy/sad/anxious?
What are you afraid of?

A sound goes off after three minutes and they change over.
The listener now becomes the speaker and speaks uninter-
rupted for three minutes.

After the sound to mark the end, they again look at each
other for one minute in silence, maybe noting how differently they think and feel about each other from the first
encounter to now.

Next, for three minutes, the players give each other feedback. Not giving advice or getting on some political platform
but how they resonated with each other's story.

When the sound goes off, they say goodbye and the game
ends.

Maybe this could be played once a day to really recognize that we're all the same. And this is my gift for world peace.

Mindfulness Exercises

I've dreamt these up to help us use tech, rather than let it use us.

1. For Phone Addiction

When standing, start to notice your breathing; the rise and fall of your chest or abdomen with each in-breath and out-breath. Notice when the mind starts its thought stream and maybe even mentally note where it's taken you. Your mind will always wander so this is simply noticing where it's gone and, without judgement or acrimony, take the focus back to the breath. This will happen again and again as the mind never stops, so congratulate yourself each time you notice and return to the breath.

When you're ready, pick up your phone and notice the feel of it in your hand; the weight, the texture. Start to walk, being aware of each movement, feeling the muscles that make walking happen. Notice the thoughts in your head, maybe how badly you want to check for messages, make a call or email. Walk to the nearest window and when you get there, open it, aware of the movements. Sense your arm lifting with the iPhone in your hand and, on an out-breath, releasing the phone through the open window. Watch as it arcs through the air and down, down, as it smashes on to the ground. Notice if you're feeling or thinking about regrets, panic or sadness. This is normal. So now slowly close the window and bring the focus back to the breath.

The above exercise can also be done facing the sea or on a balcony.

2. Urge Surfing

Maybe once a day, stop and notice when your hand automatically reaches for the phone. (If you did exercise 1, it's probably shattered. Never mind, even if it's in pieces, you'll probably reach for it anyway.) Tune in to the feelings in your body and investigate where and what 'urge' feels like. Is it in a specific area? Is it heavy or light? Does it pulse, stab, etc.? At some point, a thought will snare your attention – it could be justifying why it's urgent to make a call, or that you'll just do one call and then turn it off, or how much you hate yourself for being so desperate, or simply random thoughts. The exercise is to notice when your mind carries you away and then, gently, to take your focus to where you experienced the urge. After a few minutes, stop and notice if your feelings or thoughts have changed or not. Either way, you've done the exercise, so congratulate yourself because very few people on earth can pause before reaching for their digital drug.

Please note: a phone is a necessary tool for work, appointments or gossiping but, personally, I find myself talking for hours to people I don't even like. I created this exercise so I could have a life. Only when you've calmed your mind can you make a clear decision whether you want to talk to someone or not, or just throw it out of the window again. Now you have choice rather than a compulsion.

3. Being Present With Your Computer

At a set time when you're at your desk, send your focus to where your feet make contact with the ground, then widen the focus to the precise area where your body makes contact with the chair you're on and now widen focus again to experience the sense of your whole body. Feel your breath filling your body like a bellows, in and out. After a minute or so lift both arms, feeling their weight and the motion of moving them to lift the lid of your computer. Slowly, with awareness, lower the tips of your fingers on to the keys, sensing them through each fingertip. Watch where your thoughts go – maybe nagging you to start or finish something or maybe you're furious you're doing this exercise.

Again, take your focus to your breathing, feeling the breath filling your body like a balloon, in and out. When a thought snares you, gently take your attention back to breathing or sensing the feeling of the keys on your fingers. After a few minutes, see if anything has changed or not. Either way, you've taken a few minutes to exercise your brain, to notice your habits of rushing, and that's what breaks them.

When you go back to working and your mind is calmer, it makes it more likely you can enter that 'flow' state where the writing becomes effortless and a joy. Whenever you feel that hunched, jaw-clenched pressure to work, stop, breathe a few times into the whole body, wait and proceed with your masterpiece.

It's not our academic brilliance, talent or success that defines a great human being, it's our ability to feel compassion. We need to remind ourselves that individuals do not survive on their own. We're human because of our social connections and anything that separates us makes us less human. We need to remember how to reconnect to one another, remaking society towards human ends rather than towards the end of humans.

> 'Never doubt that a small group of thoughtful committed citizens can change the world. Indeed it is the only thing that ever has'
> – Margaret Mead

5

Food

As with many other glitches in us humans, we aren't aware of why we do what we do, and when we wake up, as from a dream, we try to blame someone else for the damage we've done to ourselves and the world. Just as we're so surprised about the climate crisis ('How did this happen? Who did this?'), we are as surprised to find we're having heart attacks and diabetes, or that one day we've woken up just plain old obese. We never think, WE DID THIS TO OURSELVES. We should all wear a T-shirt that says, 'Who can I blame?' And here's the real kicker: for the last fifty years we have known the link between health and food yet, since the 1970s, our consumption of junk food is up. You can't say you don't know about the dangers of eating crap because it's been in every newspaper, on radio, TV, tweeted, on the internet, even pictures on billboards for those who can't read.

In America, there was a campaign in 1970 that stressed that vegetables and fruit are good for you and advocated eating five a day. Ten years later they found that there had been a 3 per cent decline in the consumption of vegetables and fruit.

Similarly, we have been dumping our trash for decades and can now pay a visit to it on an island called the Great Pacific Garbage Patch, which is about 1.6 million square kilometres in size, more than double the size of Texas and three times the size of France. We don't think about where our rubbish goes when we toss it out, as if some garbage fairy comes and takes it to a magical land somewhere.

We should know though – after all, it's written about everywhere – so unless you live in a cave you have no excuse not to know. We put rubbish in our mouths, even though we now know it causes heart disease, strokes, type 2 diabetes, certain cancers, obesity and premature aging to name a few. And many of these happen to younger people; you could lose forty-five years of life compared with people who eat healthy food. Heart disease alone is responsible for 50 per cent of deaths in America. Maybe we could count the number of those who died of heart disease and compare it to the amount of burgers sold at the golden arches. All this for a taste sensation that lasts maybe ten seconds or however long it takes for you to chew and swallow. But we know what we're like because we've been here before.

When cigarette companies started putting pictures of coffins and foetuses with an X through them on the packets, the sales of tobacco actually went up. This is because when we are full of fear our rational brain closes shop and we reach for a cigarette. Remember, we do also have the capacity to use our higher brains, to pull in the reins to control the lower reptilian brain. So if the bad news has a numbing effect on us so that we are deliberately blind and deaf to warnings, maybe a book about good news will persuade people to change.

Now is the time to give you a short but completely accurate history of food.

History of Food

In the beginning, our ancient ancestors just picked from the all-you-can-eat buffet we call earth. We hunted a buffalo here, picked a berry there; nature was not disturbed at all and gave freely, regenerating itself. Everything worked in perfect harmony. Our ancestors did not think about whether food was healthy or not. Food was food and if a mushroom was poisonous so be it. Then maybe they got lazy and didn't want to move around all day for food (like me, I don't see the point of wasting my day cooking and shopping for food so I order in) and as there was no delivery service, they had to start farming.

Sometime between 3500–550 BC, Mesopotamia was the 'place to be', like Ibiza is now or was ten minutes ago. Hunting and gathering had worked fine for tribes of around 150 but with a growing population it would be a car crash; all those people trying to pick from the same trees which would be stripped bare in minutes. So in order to survive, they got the farmers (the ones who stopped moving) to grow enormous amounts of food for a burgeoning population. The farmers discovered scratching up the soil to plant the many seeds. Nature now began to be gradually depleted by ploughing and overgrazing. The ecosystem, which is the biology of soil (all the microscopic creatures and mycelia where the nutrients are), in the farmed areas of these dry nations began to collapse.

On the other hand, no plough, no civilization; we needed to plant stuff otherwise we'd starve. If a city or town ran out of food because their crop failed, they had no option but to declare war on the next-door town or city to get some. David Montgomery, in his book *Dirt*, said that all civilizations back then ended because the land that fed everyone became so degraded that people either had to move, conquer new territory or starve.

Meanwhile back in Mesopotamia (modern Syria and Iraq), they had to think of ways of preserving food. In 1200ish BC someone thought, 'I know, let's put the food in the sun to dry,' and it caught on. A simple idea but it worked. You spread out your food in the sun which evaporates the water, and *voilà*, dried food. Around the same time they also started using other ways to stop food from rotting or poisoning people. In the town square, you'd see them carrying sticks of hanging, salted fish on strings (they could also be used for decoration).

Between 3000–550 BC, when pharaohs and their queens were buried in the pyramids they had big farewell parties where friends and family buried jewellery and food for the afterlife (you know how hungry you get once you're dead?). At that time, to preserve the food, they salted it and it ended up lasting longer than they did. When they opened the tombs the pharaohs were all mummified, looking like biltong, while the food was still in great shape.

By the way, around this time (probably because they needed to eat and had run low on meat and fish) suddenly the Egyptians all went on a low-fat, high-carb diet because wholegrain and cereals became the 'It Girls' of food. Everyone started eating bread, thinking it was nourishing, but instead of getting healthier, they got sicker, smaller and fatter, their teeth rotted and their lifespan halved. We always think they were so smart; they weren't.

In 500 BC, the Greeks thought of preserving food inside jars of honey; thus the first jelly ('jam' to some of you) was born. That was their final gift to us after giving us arts, sports, medicine, law, language, science, maths and philosophy, before they collapsed.

Wars over territories were won and lost and hungry people looted and pillaged from other people's farms – you've seen the films, I don't need to spell it out. By the way, war is often instigated by hunger (not, as many believe, because of colour, race or religion but just for wanting dinner and wanting it bad). If you've seen *Joseph and the Amazing Techni-color Dreamcoat* you'll know that Joseph had a dream where he was warned that famine was coming so he advised the Pharaoh to take advantage of the boom time and stock up with food. My point is, if they'd all had refrigeration in those ol' biblical days, Joseph wouldn't have sung that song and you never would have heard of the show.

All they had was ice (which was not much use in warmer regions). In the Book of Proverbs we have proof that the Jews used ice to cool their beverages rather than to preserve their food – they had great priorities.

Scroll On a Thousand Years . . .

In the 1700s various people (including Benjamin Franklin) experimented with how to cool and freeze by a process of evaporation and by 1866 Sir Joe Fridge (that may not have been his name) invented refrigeration as we know it and meat could now be transported and traded around the world. Hurrah! (And also not hurrah as refrigeration is one of the biggest causes of CO_2 emissions.)

Meanwhile, in 1809, canning had started. Napoleon rewarded Nicolas Appert for inventing the process of preserving food in vacuum-packed glass. He thought this would be the magic answer to feeding his army, who he believed 'marched on their stomach'. The theory went, 'If you feed them, they will kill.'

Fast forward to the twentieth century. By the 1920s nobody ate. All the flappers wanted to have those boyish fig-ures which were the craze so to help them lose their hunger they smoked Lucky Strike cigarettes. An ad at the time read, 'Reach for a Lucky instead of a sweet'. So no food was really necessary during these wild and crazy bootlegger times and you didn't really need to worry about preservatives as they lived on diet pills, chewing gum and laxatives. There were rumours that the 'flappers' swallowed pills containing tapeworm eggs. Along with the weight loss, apparently, they would get diarrhoea, nausea and a fever. I don't know what this diet was called, maybe the 'Tapeworm egg, diarrhoea, nausea diet'. It would be a huge bestseller. This continued to be a slimming aid; the famous opera singer Maria Callas was rumoured to have swallowed tapeworms to lose weight.

In the 1930s, during the Great Depression, people became thrifty (when they weren't starving) so along came the cheap food brigade like Colonel Sanders from Kentucky. He decided to make chicken out of God knows what and flavoured it with his secret ingredient sprinkled on top before frying the fuck out of it; KFC was born.

During the rationing of the Second World War, convenience foods came on the market, i.e. instant coffee and cake mix. Everything was available in powder form, making it light for soldiers to carry. Very important during warfare.

By the way, after the war there was all this leftover nitrogen from explosives and bombs that were no longer needed. So farmers (remember them?) were encouraged to use it for fertilizer to speed up the growth of plants. Before that, they'd had to make do with various excreta from animals; now they added nitrogen into the mix which is still sprinkled on soil today.

The 1950s were a low point for American cuisine. Women were sick of making dishes from scratch so ready-made meals became available. Electric fridges and stoves promised to make life easier for housewives so they had more time for hoovering and doing laundry. What's odd for many of us (me) is that as we get more and more kitchen equipment and appliances, we cook less and less. We watch more cooking shows than we do cooking. I know of people who watch *Bake Off* and don't even listen, they just go up and lick the screen.

They were adding preservatives by the shovelful and no one seemed to mind. Nick Barnard, who started the Rude Health food company, explained this to me: 'If you try to give food an unnaturally long shelf life, it will give you an unnaturally short human life.'

By the late 1950s, some mad chemist invented ultra-processed food. For this he used such delicacies as (look on the back of your packets and jars): sodium nitrate, azodicar-bonamide (used in bagels – well, I'm a goner, I practically snort them), potassium bromate, propylglate monosodium glutamate, high fructose corn syrup, aspartame, soy protein isolate. The result of this cocktail, Nick told me, is known now as 'edible food-like substance'; its ingredients are mainly artificial. My grandmother would have no idea what she was looking at; hydrolysed soy protein and autolysed yeast could just as well be aliens.

And there followed Wonder Bread, Reese's Peanut Butter Cups, Popsicle and Kool-Aid (I was raised on all these, this is probably why I am five feet tall and mentally unbalanced). Lastly, I need a moment of silence for my favourite child-hood food of all, Aunt Jemima pancakes.

My Story

When I was a small girl in Evanston, Illinois, every Sunday my family would go to Aunt Jemima's pancake house – everyone in town did. We would order piles of pancakes under a mountain of bacon and maple syrup. The sign outside was a lit-up image of Aunt Jemima, a smiling African-American woman with a red chequered bandana on her head. In the 1970s it was outlawed to use this image. So (I swear to God this is true) they removed the bandana and put a big brown spot on her nose and changed the name nationally to The Brown Bear. Only in America.

Maybe a particle of what makes us keep eating dangerous food stuff is we remember it with nostalgia from our happy childhood days and when you meet someone else from your era who ate the same crap as you, it bonds you. If I meet someone who ate a Twinkie, I feel almost related. And Joanna, my editor, gets all misty-eyed when she talks about spaghetti hoops, Bird's Instant Whip and Curly Wurlys. In Australia they will hump you if you mention Tim Tam biscuits.

Nothing is sacred any more, not even bread. In bakeries and supermarkets it's processed, even when it claims to be 'multi-seed' or 'wholemeal' and all homey like mama made straight from the oven (not my mother). People have become gluten intolerant because of processed bread.

When bread was untampered with and milled with an old stone, it was made using 100 per cent of the original grain, which was fermented or sprouted. It was full of nutrients, easier to digest and reduced your chances of chronic diseases, as opposed to giving you them. But now that same loaf is stuffed full of maltodextrin, dextrose, lactose, soluble or insoluble fibre, hydrogenated interesterified oil, foaming gels and glazing agents.

Even Jesus couldn't have turned the processed bread into bread-bread. And, sorry, folks, but worse still for us than bread is cereal.

Yes, I know . . . we all had it for breakfast growing up and were told it was good for us, but we now know that Corn

Flakes and Frosties are full of salt and sugar, which are numbers one and two in breakfast killers. So much for putting tigers in our tanks.

Puffed Rice Sounds Cute But is a Killer

Puffed rice, you may be interested to know, was invented by Alexander P. Anderson. He experimented for many years and eventually in 1901 heated starch granules that were sealed in a glass tube, then smashed the glass, and the resulting explosion produced puffed rice. He became a hero of breakfast cereal and was made the face of Quaker Oats. His discovery really took off at the 1904 St Louis World Fair. Anderson brought eight bronze cannons, loaded them with six pounds of raw rice and applied heat. A blizzard of puffed rice showered the crowds, who squealed with delight.

They didn't know then that these high carbohydrate foods, when mixed with sugar and milk, are stored as fat in the body, and starting the day with these cereals will set up a craving for another high-carb dose, and a vicious cycle of overeating begins. Also, if you're not already gluten intolerant, this stuff will really get you there. (I had no idea Tony the Tiger was a drug pusher.)

Main Monster on the Table

Sugar is now considered one of the most toxic ingredients in the Western diet.

A little more bad news . . . sorry, then I'll stop.

- A study where over 430,000 people were involved in a research trial found that sugar consumption contributes to oesophageal cancer, lung cancer and bowel cancer.

- Women who consumed sweet buns and cookies more than three times a week were more likely to develop certain cancers (e.g. breast).
- Also, don't even think about sugar substitutes, they cause cancer in rats and if you're a rat that's bad news.
- Salt is bad for you too, oh, and potato chips and most fruit juices.

Once you get a hit of sugar in your bloodstream, it signals dopamine to be released in your brain which, like all drugs of choice, bangs up your craving for more. So a little sugar is okay but it's addictive, like all good things. (No one gets addicted to kale.) When they talk about sugar they keep going on about glucose, so for those of you, like me, who have no idea about these things, here's an explanation that you too can google.

When you digest food in your stomach, the carbohydrates (sugar and starches) break down into glucose. Then the stomach and small intestines absorb the glucose and release it into the bloodstream. (So far it's a good thing because we need glucose for energy.) However, in order for all this to go smoothly we have to make enough insulin (what your pancreas secretes to break down sugar) to store glucose for future use. Think of insulin like a tiny storekeeper (I picture a woman called Wendy, in sensible shoes) who keeps your blood sugar from getting too high. If your body stops producing enough insulin or your cells become resistant to it, it can cause diabetes. It still doesn't end there . . .

When you eat excess sugar, the extra insulin in your bloodstream can inflame the walls of your arteries that run throughout your body. They get thicker and stiffer, which damages your heart and, over time, leads to heart disease, heart failure, strokes, etc.

In the old prehistoric days we chased our dinner so we could eat what we needed fatwise; now we sit for a living and there lies the rub – we get fat. (Also, things like trans fat didn't grow on trees back then.)

Trans fats, patented in 1903, occur in hydrogenated vegetable oil. Adding hydrogen atoms (bombing food) to cooking oils created saturated fats that helped goodies stay moist and chewy longer with a longer shelf life. Crisco was the first company to develop this technique (which is another product I was weaned on), but now it's banned. Since the 1980s the results of various trials have shown that trans fats were linked to heart attacks and that cholesterol was hardly affected by cutting fat out of the diet, but in an age where the industry was at its most powerful, consumers weren't informed of this!

In 2000, the US Food and Drug Administration (FDA) released a report estimating that about 7,000 deaths a year could be prevented by removing trans fat from margarine and other foods. And later, in 2001, a report confirmed that trans fat was associated with heart disease. We had no way of distinguishing between polyunsaturated fats, which are healthy, and trans fats. For more than a century hydrogenated oil had been seen as a magic ingredient that gave food freshness and crispiness and then, overnight, it was banned by law. So suddenly it has disappeared, no apology, no nothing. Thank God the younger generation demand more transparency than older consumers, who just bought what they saw on TV. (I thought there really was a leprechaun living in my Lucky Charms cereal and I'd still be buying Crisco if it hadn't been banned. I used to use it as moisturizer when I wasn't eating it. Who knew?)

Back to Food

From the 1950s on, it was less about what food people ate and more what they didn't eat because slimming diets now dictated our food choice, not how healthy or good it tasted. In 1953 the American biochemist Ancel Keys thought that the fat in our diet increased our cholesterol levels and that's why we got heart disease. The theory was that fat clogged your arteries like grease poured down the drain. Everyone bought into this until . . .

In 1972 the book *Dr Atkins' Diet Revolution* came out and tens of millions of people ate it up. This kick-started the modern high-fat/low-fat debate. His *New Diet Revolution* became even more popular, mainly because celebrities went on it. And people eat what famous people eat – maybe they think that if they have the same food in their gullets, they'll be famous too.

Dr Atkins started the new thinking: that a high-carb, low-fat diet wouldn't make you lose weight or keep you healthy and insisted that high-fat, low-carb diets are the way to keep trim and alive.

He was inspired by William Banting, a prosperous London undertaker and self-published author of 'Letter on Corpulence' (you won't find his work on Amazon so don't even look), who way back in 1862 started a new diet. He was overly portly and was told by his doctor that rather than nix out the fat, to eat as much of it as he could but cut out sugar, sweets, potatoes and other carbs. He not only lost weight but his cholesterol levels dropped and he became a convert.

I was told throughout my life that fats were taboo and now, it turns out, that was a lie. So many wasted years tossing away egg yolks, cutting the fat off meat, and now we're supposed to snort fat. Trials were done and no matter how much fat volunteers ate, their cholesterol levels weren't affected. Turns out the body lowers its own levels when it has enough.

Banting's diet was based on the rich-in-fat diet our ancestors ate to survive in the distant past. This storing of the fat gave them tremendous amounts of energy to run at high speeds for long distances, as they chased antelopes and lions. (These days, people in Wisconsin can't even get out of their chairs. Times have changed.)

Banting had quite a following at the time but for some reason the diet fizzled out and completely disappeared by the end of the Second World War, at which point, for some reason, it became excluded from the medical books and replaced by the low-fat, high-carb diet, maybe because farmers got huge state subsidies, therefore making a large profit from feeding us the same crap they were feeding to cows.

There Followed Craze After Craze

In 1981 we got the Beverly Hills Diet giving people a six-week food-combining regimen and turning Judy Mazel into a Hollywood diet guru. She gave us the idea that we should eat a lot of fat-burning pineapple. That for ten days you could only eat fruit then gradually other foods were introduced. So many people, including the famous, got the runs. Liza Minnelli embraced the diet and became a stick insect almost overnight.

The Sleeping Beauty Diet came somewhere in this time, based on an idea that when a person is sleeping, they are not eating (duh). The advocates of this diet use sedatives to go to sleep during the day to avoid consuming food. Elvis Presley for one used this method; for several days he went into a medically induced coma in an attempt to lose weight.

Michael Jackson seemed to also be on this diet for other reasons than weight loss.

My Story

There followed more and more diets that worked less and less. I went on one where I ate only grapefruit and ended up in hospital having the pulp removed from my stomach. Not long ago, I went big time into the juicing diet. Whole gardens were pulverized in my blender. I almost exploded while on a train, I was so sick. I had been drinking my flask of vegetables like water; someone told me later I had drunk the equivalent of four football fields filled with broccoli.

Now, foods are labelled with the words 'healthy', 'organic', 'eco-friendly' as if nature is going to say, 'Look! Ruby's eating an eco-friendly chocolate bar, that's going to stop the ice cap melting. Thank you, Ruby.' I recently saw in LA a few 'organic' nail bars; I wasn't planning on eating my nails, I just wanted them clipped. My favourite diet that I've heard about is the Breatharian Diet where no food is involved, you just breathe. Again in LA, someone told me about a Breatharian Restaurant. Imagine the profit margin!

Fasting took off in 2012 but is still popular today and I'm not talking about people in countries with no food. Maybe it is so embraced in the West because it's not just cheap, it's free. It's sometimes known as the 5.2 diet; you eat normally for five days then restrict calories to 500 for women (which is about half a breadstick) and 600 for men, on two non-consecutive days. There are claims it can reduce the risk of cancer and heart disease and that you can live past a hundred.

Starving seems to work based on the fact that when your body realizes there is no food incoming (in other words, zero calories), your body calls a code-red emergency and raids your fat stores to keep you alive.

Now once your body has emptied the cupboard (after about two days) it switches on an emergency source of energy – the ketonic system. Ketosis will power your body for days, because this system is designed to get us through famine or being in a state of fight or flight. It's an emergency generator so your brain actually works better when it is operating. The body is now in a state of autophagy (Greek for eating itself). The good news about eating yourself means your insulin levels have hit the dust, so you'll be free of diabetes, heart disease and high cholesterol but you may be dead.

The Banting Diet had a resurgence a few years ago in the disguise of the Paleo Diet except with this one there's no carbs. Just fat.

Vegetarianism/Veganism

The Buddha, Gandhi, Bernard Shaw and Shelley were all advocates of living without meat so it's been going for a while and can hardly be described as a health fad. And now there's evidence that meat is unsustainable partly because farmers have to take up huge tracts of land to grow maize or wheat, purely to feed animals and not us. Also, animals are cute and our friends and who wants to eat a friend? Vegetarians don't eat pigs, chickens, cows or fish (some cheat and eat fish but don't tell anyone).

The story goes that in 1944 a small group of vegetarians broke away from the Vegetarian Society of England and formed the Vegan Society. (I'm wondering if there was a war between them? I want to be a member of both sides immediately.) Vegans (named from the first and last letters of vegetarian) choose not to consume dairy, eggs or any other products of animal origin because they don't want to see them suffer but also for ethical, health and environmental reasons. They believe going plant-based reduces the risk of heart disease, type 2 diabetes, cancer and premature death.

There are nutritional problems being discovered with this new vegan processed food that you see in the supermarkets as they have lots of additives and are often sugary or full of salt, so the jury is out on how healthy the diet is. The worry is that many vegans eat chips, biscuits and ready-made meals pumped full of chemicals and saturated fats. These are not healthier than their meat-filled alternatives despite the marketing, as they are still processed.

Tim Spector advocates choosing healthy food (that includes whatever food you most enjoy) and cutting down on meat and dairy is probably a good idea for the environment so being a part-time vegan (or flexitarian) ensures you don't become deficient in things like vitamin B12.

Michael Pollan, one of the main influencers on diet, says that most of what we eat now is not food; it was he who named it 'food-like substance' and said that we should follow his maxim: 'Eat food, not too much, mostly plants.' The vegetarian/vegan global market was worth $51 billion in 2016 and has leapt to $140 billion in just four years. Money talks and now, whatever the reservations of the food gurus, it's the coolest thing to be vegan. You cannot be a hipster without it. I've tried – even with a fake beard I can't pass.

Okay, this is why so many of us are driven insane. Have you noticed that every diet I've discussed has groupies who insist that theirs is the key to the kingdom of healthiness? One week I can eat an egg, the next week I'm told it's like dropping an A-bomb on my innards. Is cholesterol a good witch or a wicked witch? The Atkins Diet tells me to swallow whole herds, vegans would rather kill me than a chicken. Butter? Cookies? Cancer or what? WHO DO WE BELIEVE? EVERYONE CAN'T BE RIGHT!

Enter Probiotics – Very Good News

Again, everything I believed in the past has been turned on its head. I haven't eaten an egg since I was thirty-two because I was told I'd have a heart attack (unless I just ate the white part and chucked the poison part, the yolk). Now I'm told an egg a day makes you live to 106 and gives you nice hair.

It's the same when I hear the word 'bacteria'; I was under the impression that it was something that needed to be scraped, soaped or deodorized immediately. Turns out microbes, meaning bacteria, yeasts and fungi, are all over us, inside and out, and are running the show. There are trillions and trillions of tiny living things in our eyes, ears, nose and other crevices but mostly in our gastrointestinal tract, all of them making sure we keep on ticking.

I found out about the importance of microbes from an interview I did with Tim Spector, one of the world's great gut gurus, for my Audible series *No Brainer*. He says, 'The state of our gut biome affects our physical and psychological health.' Apparently, microbes help us fight cancer, digest food, turn what we eat into B2 and B12, and control our moods by changing what happens chemically inside of us. (They don't know for sure yet, but depression just might be influenced by activity in the gut rather than the brain.) Microbes are like the Wizard of Oz behind the curtain, running us.

We are all part of a planet full of these things. Don't get

grossed out, they are keeping you alive. Now they tell us, instead of washing our hands, we should stick them in soil because dirt is our best friend. Things like gardening (which I'm allergic to) are a wonderful bacteria-picker-upper and when the baby drops its dummy, don't grab it in mid-air or sterilize it, let it drop on the ground so the baby acquires an army of microscopic crawly things to build up the immune system. Tim told me that babies get natural microbes from the mother during that trip (agonizing for the mother) down the birth canal. If they're born through caesarean section (as mine were), the kids have more chance of getting allergies and more problems with weight, later in life. This is why in some hospitals, when a woman has a caesarean, they often rub vaginal fluids on the baby to compensate for the lack of bacteria. It's called swabbing. I asked him if it was too late to swab my son. Tim asked how old my son was, I said thirty; there was a long silence.

I asked him to recommend a practitioner who would analyse the state of my gut. He put me in touch with Miguel Toribio-Mateas, a nutritionist who is also a clinical neuroscientist, specializing in probiotics and mental health. Tim told me he was the top nutritionist for testing and manipulating my gut biome. Here's the bad news: you have to somehow get your faeces into a small tube which is one of the more horrible experiences in my life. I won't give you the details but using a spoon or shoehorn doesn't work. Anyway, you send your samples away (imagine if they went to the wrong address what the receiver would think) and then, a few weeks later, Miguel gives you the results of your gut condition.

Miguel told me our gut bacteria share information with the rest of the body by producing molecules that work a bit like Wi-Fi. These signals from the gut are picked up by different systems around the body, which form a kind of information-sharing network, making minute adjustments as a result. He told me that in your gut microbiome there are opportunistic bacteria (the not-so-friendly guys) probing your immune system which, to defend itself, is learning and changing all the time. The microbiome is a collection of living organisms, communicating the whole time with your immune system; telling it to attack or not to attack. Around 70 per cent of your immune system is in your gut. In fact, the thin layer of mucus that protects your gut lining is the bit which picks up information from gut bugs, translating it into messages that give instructions to various parts of the immune system to become active and fight. Different foods activate or deactivate these messages by feeding different gut bugs.

The thinking is that in order to keep our gut biome healthy, we need to eat food that feeds beneficial or health-promoting bacteria. You need to look at your biome as a team of different gut bugs working together and the aim is to make the team more efficient.

Luckily, my faeces went to the right address so Miguel called me to report on the diversity of my biome. I had an average diversity of bacteria for a person in the UK, but higher than average in America; meaning they are less healthy over there, gut-wise. He suggested a fibre-rich, Mediterranean-style, 'rainbow-coloured' diet, with plenty of probiotic foods, largely based on Tim's book, *The Diet Myth*, and said he'd test me again after six weeks.

Probiotic Foods

Probiotics are living organisms found in foods such as natural yogurt, kefir (fermented milk), cheese (especially with blue veins – which are caused by probiotic fungi), raw milk, kombucha (fermented tea), algae, kimchi (fermented cabbage, often hot/spicy). You probably guessed that fermented is good for you; I used to think it was like eating acid and would give me ulcers. Wrong again.

The more diverse your microbes, the more different chemicals they can produce to protect you. Miguel told me to eat as many different foods as possible, meaning as many different-coloured vegetables and fruit. Oh, more good news, certain natural chemicals are like rocket fuel for microbes, they have funky names (like polyphenols and flavanols) and they're trapped in the bright pigments that make berries blue, red or pink. They're also in coffee and dark (over 70 per cent) chocolate. I can eat chocolate, how happy am I on this diet?

This gut biome theory is in its infancy but so far medical and scientific evidence shows that it's a highly accurate system of testing our health as it involves looking at the whole picture. We have 20,000 genes that determine who we are, but we have around 20 million bacterial genes, so from that point of view, you're about 99 per cent bacterial and not quite 1 per cent you. It's difficult to change genes but you can change the composition of your microbes immediately, by eating the right foods. And because we still don't know for certain which foods are best, eating a rainbow of brightly coloured fruit and veg every day is your best bet.

Good News for the Future of Food

There is a change in the air – over the last few years many people have voted with their feet and started programmes and initiatives to prevent waste and promote better quality food. Twenty years ago, councils were putting up posters to encourage people to take an allotment and grow their own vegetables, now there is usually a five-year waiting list.

Gardening groups and allotments are blooming and, along with cooking, crafting, sewing and repairing stuff, there are TV shows all day to get your fix of planting stuff. Recently, too, organizations like the Skip Garden have started to create urban spaces where people can grow veg and who also organize pot-luck suppers where you bring your own contributions and make a banquet together.

Everyone is now getting the connection between what you eat and whether it is healthy for you – even if knowing it is all, it's still better than wolfing down stuff without realizing it's harmful as we have been for so many years; give us time and we'll get there.

These Beacons of Hope are the people who are regenerating landscapes, enhancing livelihoods and restoring people's health and well-being; not just in their own backyards but globally (because they care about the world these days). Here are a few examples (I wish we had thought of these rather than wolfing burgers):

London Grows, an initiative funded by the Mayor of London, encourages Londoners to get outside and grow stuff, with the aim of re-establishing local gardens as communal hubs. They're helping run hundreds of fruit, vegetable and herb gardens around the capital and hopefully will be extended nationwide soon.

The People's Fridge – better known as Freddie – is just one example of several social projects carried out by Impact Hub Brixton. Their aim is to provide a place for locals and businesses to deposit their surplus food and make the food available, for free, to anyone who wants it. There is an actual fridge on the street full of food and anyone can help themselves.

The Orchard Project In the UK we import most of the fruit we eat so local orchards have been in a state of decline since the 1950s. A mere banana has to travel 50,000 miles to get into your mouth. In the UK there's a group of food-savvy people who are busy training community leaders in nurturing communal orchards all over the country; they can share out the fruit and pass on that knowledge to anyone interested in getting involved.

This change in the air isn't just happening here, it's happening globally.

Zero Budget Natural Farming In Andhra Pradesh, India, there are already 180,000 farmers who have joined this government-backed, chemical-free programme that promotes traditional farming processes so that everyone isn't so hooked on processed foods sold by the giant supermarkets and they keep their jobs. They're using a system where knowledge and skills are shared through farmer-to-farmer mentoring. They plan to scale this up to 6 million farmers by 2024.

Community Markets for Conservation (COMACO) is a Zambian scheme to retrain poachers to be farmers. 'Skilling farmers in agroecological approaches helps generate an alternative income and livelihood to the (illegal) hunting of wildlife.'

EOSTA is based in the Netherlands and produces and imports sustainable, organic and fair-trade fruits and vegetables. It gives the consumer a full report of what the true costs of their products are and this builds trust between the growers and the eaters.

Farmers Markets have already made their mark and are now a worldwide phenomenon. This is a great indicator that people are starting to care about food being local. In America there are more than 6,000 farmers markets, which is a 50 per cent increase since 1994 . . . so that's better than a kick in the ass.

Food Waste

Food production has the single greatest man-made environmental impact on the planet. What's more, wasted food, if it were a country, would rank as the third largest emitter of greenhouse gases after China and the US. How about them apples (which now come from Venezuela)?

But coming to the rescue is a food campaign group called Feedback who have been researching this phenomenon and have come up with some solutions.

Feedback has found that farmers waste around 16 per cent of their crop before it even leaves the field or barn because the produce is not the right shape or size for supermarket tastes. So they have started a Gleaning Network. (Gleaning is an archaic word for gathering the leftover grain in the field after harvest.) This gives volunteers an opportunity to engage with the food system hands-on by rescuing fresh, surplus fruit and veg (which is just bent out of shape) from farms where it would otherwise be wasted, and get it to people's plates.

Their research also shows that the problem here is not just the misshapen veg but lies with the chains of supermarkets which dominate the food market and control the farmers' livelihoods. The main issue is that they can't be specific enough about how much they need so they set up orders with farms but then, if the demand fluctuates (maybe it's raining and they don't need so many strawberries), they simply pull the plug on the grower, who is left with a shed of mouldy fruit.

A conservative estimate of farm-level food waste is 2.5 million tonnes, representing a lost produce value of £0.8 billion (*The Grocer*, 2017). This is why there is pressure now on supermarkets to sell wonky-shaped veg and to buy more local food. With the increased numbers of farmers markets, let's hope the future is 'farm to fork' food.

Which is a good way to lead into talking about what is new and exciting in the farming world.

Farming: Where the Food Comes From

I've already mentioned that since the end of the Second World War there has been a massive increase in cereal being grown industrially because it was vital we could 'feed the nation'. Farmers were encouraged to tear out the hedges separating their fields and make room for the enormous new machines which were going to revolutionize the production of food.

When the farmers needed to plant acres of the wheat, maize and barley that make up cereal, they had to add chemicals to kill the large amounts of weeds. Genetic engineering also came in to 'improve' the crop, making it resistant to various weeds and pests but also making the plants toxic.

When you continually add pesticides, there are chemical reactions that burn off the soil, and as it degrades, it becomes harder and harder to work so you need heavier ploughs which damage the soil even more. Eventually it's transformed into clay or sand (creating deserts). In the last twenty years an area the size of France has been made barren this way.

These ploughs churned up the soil, breaking the topsoil,

which is known as the skin of the planet, releasing huge amounts of CO_2 into the air. A third of all man-made CO_2 has been released this way. (The world's ploughed soils have lost over 50 per cent of their original carbon.) Ploughing also damages the biodiversity in the soil, which is nature's way of supplying different nutrients for the soil to be healthy. In one tablespoon, there are more creatures than there have ever been humans walking on the earth and 98 per cent of the genetic diversity of land-based life.

John Cherry, a regenerative farmer, told me: 'We can massively reduce global warming by capturing carbon dioxide from the air using living plants. It's really simple and it happens really fast. All you have to do is keep the soil covered at all times by having living plants growing and not disturbing it. Undisturbed plants growing in healthy soil take in high amounts of CO_2 from the air and put it back into the ground. Because there's so much of it, farmland has the potential to store far more than the world's forests. So farming in this way means we don't need new tech to remove CO_2 from air; to prevent more climate change we just need to restore earth's green carpet.'

There's a movement going on now which recognizes that ploughing and intensive farming is not good for the health of the soil or what's growing in it. The less you meddle with the soil, the more it thrives with all its microscopic life that adds nutrients to whatever you're growing. So if you farm as though you are copying nature instead of controlling it, you're going to grow the healthiest possible plants.

John added: 'The good news is that it can be restored to health in a matter of a few years and it can also be turned into a carbon-capturing sink. So land that was leaking carbon into the air can recover and act like a carbon sponge to soak it back up again.'

Healthy Soil – Healthy Food

John and a growing number of forward-thinking farmers are part of a new movement called Regenerative Agriculture where you can plant crops without ploughing up the soil. They've invented 'no-till' machines which plant the seeds straight into the ground without disturbing it.

For regenerating the soil, these are the golden rules:

- Keep the soil covered with living matter (stubble, plants, manure)
- Plant many different things in it, not one crop
- Never plant the same thing you did last year (each plant adds a different nutrient to the soil)
- And wean your soil off the fungicides, herbicides and pesticides (the soil will heal itself)

Humans and the Humus are Connected

Every animal, plant and microorganism is full of bacteria. In the soil, they beaver away, making sure plants stay healthy by fighting off harmful enemies and keeping the atmosphere and earth stable. In humans, bacteria also declare war on invading microbes, and keep us stable inside. Bacteria are everywhere, from the moon (yes, some were found on the lens of a camera someone left there) to about 100 trillion tonnes of them below our feet; meaning there is probably more life under the earth than on top of it (so much for feeling you're special).

In between each and every plant, there's a web of fungus and mitochondria that works as a kind of answering- and room-service system. So if a fern gets sick because, for example, it's dying from lack of nitrogen, it sends out SOS signals to other plants through its roots, like broadband, and some plant far away will pick up the message and send the exact formula of nutrients the sick fern needs to flourish. What's incredible is that they don't just help their own species; the soil web doesn't care or know which plants it's helping.

What goes for the soil, goes for us. The new thinking is that when we reduce our microbes through eating less diverse food or killing them with things like antibiotics, we become unwell. Similarly, when we kill off microbes and insects in the soil (which break down organic matter while supplying and distributing nutrients), we're destroying the earth and what we eat.

We are related to the earth, biologically. If you put one of our cells and a fungal cell from the soil under a microscope, they're nearly the same. In South Africa they found mycelium infused in the lava from 1.4 billion years ago. Think about it, we're only separated from fungi by a mere 650 million years and they've had their form longer than we've had ours by about a billion years. Fungi was there before us and will be there long after we're gone.

Understanding that we're connected to the earth, we need to become aware of how we treat it. Daniel Goleman in his book *Ecological Intelligence* says:

> We need to recognize the hidden web of connections between human activity and nature's systems and the subtle complexities of their interaction. So we need to be vigilant about monitoring our behaviour in commerce and industry as well as our individual actions and behaviours and how they interact with nature; that's ecological intelligence. If we keep alert to all of this, then we will see interconnections

between our actions and their hidden impact on planet health and social systems.

I realize that all the green shoots I've discovered from writing this book really stem from similar beliefs; we are waking up and finding ways 'to connect human activity to the larger flow of nature'.

6

World Savers

In this final chapter I'm going to pick out a few initiatives created by the actual people who plant the seeds from which the green shoots grow. To be clear, I'm aware there are hundreds of thousands of groups and individuals passionately and selflessly helping or healing but I've chosen these few because they remind me of who I was when I was young and had their spark. These people have the same expression I had in my eyes when I was eighteen. I've said that this book is to make me feel better and just being near people who radiate compassion allows me to bask in their heat. Love is catching, as is hate, but I chose them and their grassroot movements because I know they're the real deal. They loosened the hold I had on my own self-obsession and allowed me to become part of the world. I can see why they glow – there is nothing as high-making as helping someone.

My Story

In 1969 I was in Chicago for the Democratic Convention. I lied about my age (you had to be over eighteen) to get a job working for the democratic nominee, Gene McCarthy. I was staying in the headquarters at the Chicago Hilton for the convention and one night, looking out of the window on to State Street, I saw a line-up of tanks with guns erect, rumbling their way towards the hotel from both directions. I recall turning to people inside, telling them that Otto Preminger (big Hollywood director at the time) must be directing a war movie because why else would there be tanks coming down State Street? I was wrong. They were coming for us. Across the street from the hotel was Grant Park which had turned into a political Woodstock, filled with sixties revolutionaries, shouting anti-war speeches through megaphones about fucking the establishment, banning bombs, civil rights, and chanting ditties en masse: *'Guns, bullets, gas masks, LBJ can kiss my ass'* (the current president was Lyndon B. Johnson). It was a heady confluence of people like Frank Zappa, Angela David, Abbie Hoffman and the Black Panthers, with music provided by The Grateful Dead. What's not to like? In the evenings, I'd stroll across the street to the park, thinking I was the coolest thing on earth as no one from my high school would have dared do this. That night, the party didn't stop as the tanks pulled up in front of the park. There was a lull and suddenly Chicago cops spilled out of the tanks, with clubs swinging, beating the hell out of anyone they could get their hands on as I watched from the window on the twenty-first floor. The next thing was all the elevators on our floor opened simultaneously and we were invaded. I remember being dragged by my long hair into the elevator, down to the lobby and thrown into the street, where I was greeted by circling helicopters dropping canisters of tear gas. Richard Daley was Mayor of Chicago at the time, and was known as 'the fascist pig'. He hated all things non-conformist and hippy and right here in the middle of his kingdom, he had a 15,000-strong flower-waving army from his worst nightmare, shitting on his turf. So he had called out his hounds to collect scalps.

I was totally innocent and couldn't get my head around what was happening. This was my home town, Chicago, where I went shopping with my mother to the big fancy department stores and visited my dentist, who once a month tightened my braces. Now, I was running through the streets, past Manny's Deli, Saks Fifth Avenue and Neiman Marcus, trying to get away from the fumes of tear gas, which felt like a thousand nails being hammered into my lungs. Wet handkerchiefs were handed out to put over our mouths for protection, but nothing helped.

The next day, I got into the actual convention to vote for the Democratic presidential candidate and, before my very eyes, watched the electoral college at work. The room was the size of a football stadium and we all looked down on the state representatives with their teams. Someone on stage asked each state to cast their vote for either Hubert Humphrey (warmonger) or Gene McCarthy (anti-war). At the start, it seemed pretty straightforward but very quickly they started to turn off the microphones for those states that were about to vote McCarthy. You could see people yelling but couldn't hear what they said. This meant the only votes heard were for Humphrey. I saw the headlines announcing the result in the stack of newspapers that had already been printed before the votes were in. I knew then that all those times at school I'd said, 'I pledge my allegiance to the flag of the United States of America . . .' it was a sham and it was around then, I decided, after waking up to the

> **fact my country was corrupt, I would leave the US and
> go to the UK . . . the rest is history. By the way, I was
> arrested later and my father wrote a personal letter
> to Mayor Daley, thanking him.**

For decades now, I've thought people younger than me
were asleep at the wheel, politically – personalities as bland
as milk toast, accompanied by music as bland as milk toast –
and then suddenly there's this new generation that wasn't
going to take shit any more. So some of these people are the
world savers I've chosen.

If you find the world you're living in a little distressing
or depressing, I urge you to get in touch with a group doing
something constructive in the world and join. Maybe at first go
listen, then maybe go again for longer and meet the people
involved and then take the plunge and go do some work with
them. I promise you will never have to see a shrink again. Exist-
ential crisis over. You don't have to go for the ones I've chosen,
you can hunt down your own, but don't get overwhelmed
because there are oceans of volunteer projects. Choose the
one that you resonate with because unless you feel an emotional tie you won't stick with it. If you know someone's
pain, you'll commit, and the great trade-off is that if you help
someone, you feel good, so you're helping yourself.

Here are my top four favourite world savers.

My First World Saver: Samos Refugee Camp

I don't know why but for many years I've thought about
working with refugees. Maybe because my parents were
refugees and if they hadn't made it into America, I wouldn't
be in existence and, worse, you wouldn't be reading this.

Here's how I got involved. Years ago, Juliet Stevenson (fellow thesp) told me she was driving a busful of clothes to the refugees in Calais. I remember saying even before she finished the sentence, 'I'm coming with you.'

But I didn't go and it has always niggled that I should have. So finally I called Indigo Volunteers who place volunteers with grassroots charities working in the refugee camps and told them to sign me up. The person on the phone asked where exactly I wanted to go to volunteer. I said I'd look at photos and get back to her – like I was choosing a holiday spa destination. And in that spirit, I clicked straight to Airbnb sites to find out what kind of accommodation was available. (Sometimes I disgust myself.)

There weren't many delightful Airbnbs on the refugee islands so I asked them to find me somewhere to stay. From the moment I volunteered, I saw myself as an incredibly compassionate person; tipping higher than usual and generally being less of a bitch for the next few weeks until departure. On the way to the airport, I had to take a taxi because I was carrying two extra-large suitcases, crammed with items I'd stolen from hotels over the years. I announced to the driver I was bringing all this for refugees, waiting for him to fall to his knees and hand me a Victoria Cross. At that point I wasn't aware that where I was going, they might not have a bathtub in which to drop the Hawaiian, ying-ling, patchouli and coco-infused bath bombs I brought by the dozens.

24 March 2019

EasyJet charged me four times what it would cost to go first class to the Maldives to get those two gigantine suitcases on board containing the very crucial Elemis moisturizers (all stolen) the refugees would need to survive. I landed at mid-night in Athens, then rented a car to head for the Nea Kavala camp in northern Greece. The signposts were not in English as expected. I had to go from Thessaloniki to Axioupoli to Polykastro and those aren't even written in English on a nor-mal day and now they're in fucking Greek. Who reads Greek? All at once, my Google map person started speaking to me not in Greek but with a Greek attitude, telling me to stay left but only if I felt like it and pick up some feta on the way. I drove most of the way on the hard shoulder as I like to drive on the wild side. Hours later, it had dwindled down to a dirt road, with high barbed-wire fences on both sides. I knew I was in serial killer country, especially when the road just ended at a locked fence. I'm sure I now hold the world's record for the longest driven distance in reverse to Polykas-tro. I had joined a fellow volunteer group on Facebook prior to arrival, who were all from Norway for some reason. I assumed they were from Norway because (I'm not making this up) their names were Ase and Tuird. Ase had described our hotel a month earlier to me, saying, 'It has a certain charm but during winter [which it was] they did turn off hot water . . . also no toilet paper.'

25 March 2019

I met Ase and Tuird and the woman in charge of volunteers the following morning, who briefed us about the ground rules of the camp. Nea Kavala is built on what was the local airport on a runway 1 km wide and 23 km long. Families live in single containers made of corrugated tin but we're not supposed to say container, we should call it a caravan and not to call anyone refugees, they're residents.

When you arrive, no matter how briefed you are, it's

everything you'd never expect; no matter how desolate you think this might be, it's worse. My job that morning was laundry duty with Paolo, a wild-haired, earringed South American who I'd describe as a do-gooder junkie. He 'island volunteer' hops from one refugee camp to another and, on holiday, builds dams in Nigeria. He gave me step-by-step instructions on how to collect, wash, dry and return the laundry and I fucked up on every step because I was too busy talking to everyone who handed me their bag.

One guy from Iraq told me he had a PhD in physics and his dissertation was about how, metaphysically, all people are the same; all made up of particles. This notion threatened the regime so much, they had chased him out of the country and killed his family. I just held his bag full of laundry and was unable to move.

Afterwards, I peeked into some of the container/caravans and saw large families smashed into a tin shoebox, and when they'd spot me, they'd welcome me in for coffee with big smiles. I kept thinking we're so similar, laughing about the same things, except their eyes have seen relatives and friends blown up and I've only seen it on television, which makes us universes apart.

Finally, it was time for lunch and not one of the Norwegians, not Ase or Tuird, asked me to eat with them. Paolo saw me desperately seeking a lunchmate but pretended he didn't. I know, I know, there are people here who have had to escape death, crossing the ocean on a raft, and I'm sad because no one wants to have lunch with me.

I was hating myself a lot at this moment so I drove to a local supermarket and wandered up and down the aisles, sulking and munching items from the shelves. I bumped into a refugee who asked me if I was okay. For obvious reasons, I didn't want to share my pain that Ase didn't ask me to lunch so I changed the subject, asking him if he wanted a lift back to the camp. He didn't speak English but once we set off, he indicated with violent hand signals that he found my driving terrifying. A man who risked himself crossing the sea in an inner tube tells me my driving frightens him; that's not a good review.

My afternoon job was working in the market; a big wooden storage unit filled with donated clothes where once a week people can come and pick out items, not with money but with a substitute called 'drops'. Each family is given 1,500 drops a month to spend on clothes, toothpaste, toys, etc. I'm given instructions on how many drops everything costs, how to use the cash register and how to deduct it from their credit. I fuck this job up too. I try to explain, using mime, that I'm an idiot. I'm moved to bicycle rental, which is considered the easiest job, and also fuck that up. No one is talking to me now.

26 March 2019

Yesterday, I had asked Paolo if he wanted to have dinner with me (I was completely shunned by the Norwegians). He didn't look pleased but he agreed to pick me up at my hotel at 8.00. I sat like Miss Havisham in the lobby and it was a no-show so I got a kebab and went to bed. This morning, as I was walking down the street, I was yanked out of my ruminations of self-flagellation by a Syrian boy, weaving a spiderweb of threads, who asked if he could make me a bracelet. I wanted to say, 'What for? I'm an asshole,' but he looked at me with such affection I thanked him. As he crocheted his gift, he told me when he was around eleven his family were told he had to join the military to help kill Kurds. To protect him, his parents hid him and his brother in the house for nearly four years. He slept in the day and maybe once or twice in all those years he went out in the night, but not far. Without any bitterness, when I asked him what he did all that time, he told me he helped his mother clean and took care of his baby brother, keeping him quiet so they wouldn't be detected. I'm standing in front of the Syrian version of Anne Frank. Finally, the whole family left in two separate lifeboats. He made it to Turkey and waited for a whole day on shore, gradually realizing his parents weren't coming. He was fourteen. They jailed him and gave him one potato a day for two years and from there he ended up in Nea Kavala. Finally, his family followed and they've started selling a few cans of tinned food in the camp. He told me how happy he is to be able to live in the container with all six of his family in one room and the 3' × 3' shop where he works the night shift. And this angel is making me a bracelet. I'm so not worthy.

The night before, I'd called the head of volunteers, requesting to be transferred to another refugee camp. I explained, I'm a writer and needed to see a variety of camps for the book. This was partially true but I also wanted to move to somewhere I might be more popular. Today she messaged me to meet someone later that night called Aslam. She said he knows everything that's happening in every camp and could advise me. Probably she didn't believe I was a writer but thought I was just a pain in the ass. I got to the restaurant early and there was one of the Norwegians already sitting there (who invited him?), who looked at me blankly.

Suddenly, Tuird starts talking to me, telling me an amusing story about vomiting the night before from eating bad liver. It's the first time I've heard him say a complete sentence.

Aslam arrives, with long black hair, a moustache and the eyes of a madman but a very charismatic one. He tells me he has to go outside immediately because he won't go in a restaurant that doesn't let him smoke and he smokes a hundred cigarettes a day (told to me with such pride), so eating is pretty much out for him. Before his exit, seconds after his entrance, he asks me with a 'fuck you' tone in his voice, 'What is it you want to see? People come here and look and then they go home and say, "I saw it." As if it's a brave thing to just look at it. So what you want?'

With my voice quivering, I tried to explain that I'm a writer and um . . . (I'm winging it), I write so . . . I'd like to see how everyone's doing . . . I'd like to see what's on, say, Lesvos, my friend is there and she says it's more of an emergency over there (now I'm sweating and making stuff up) . . .

He breaks in. 'And you think there's no emergency here?' I'm now becoming the idiot he thinks I am.

I say, 'Nea Kavala seems sort of orderly and in control with all the containers in rows and everything . . . um . . .'

'What you think is ordered? The women are too afraid to come out. There are rapes and knife fights, they kill each other at night; in summer they boil in the tin cans and in winter they freeze so what do you mean by it's under control? On Lesvos it's a mess but they still have a lot of hope. Here it's *ordered*' – he spits that word out at me – 'but there is no hope. There is nowhere to go from here, it's a prison. In Lesvos, they dream of coming here or to Europe, where if you're caught, the authorities will pick you up and throw you out and you're back here.'

I say, 'Like snakes and ladders?' He really hates me.

From this point on, everything I say, Aslam says the opposite; even when I say exactly what he just said, he opposes me, getting angrier and angrier.

My voice is now a squeak. He has been with me an hour and it feels like years. He finally tells me if I want to see what refugee camps look like I should look on Google, and leaves. At the end of the table were two women I hadn't noticed before. I heard them talking about going to Samos (another island) the next day. Before I could get control of my mouth, I said, 'I'm coming with you.' They were thrilled at my enthusiasm and spontaneity, so agreed. Tuird looked relieved and I detected a smile.

27 March 2019

I met Holly and Molly (my new friends from the restaurant) at the airport. Aslam was also there again, who looked shocked and pissed off when he saw me.

The small plane was flown by a blind person. No one can hit the ground that hard knowing where it is. It turned out that Aslam and I were staying in the same hotel and in the taxi there I told him again that I was a writer and needed to witness with my own eyes what was going on to write about it. Looking on Google wasn't the idea so I'd like to go into the camp. Now he was incandescent, saying I couldn't just swan in there and see what I wanted to see, it had to be set up by agencies months in advance for permissions. No one could just show up and see a camp. I told him to wait and see. Just watch me.

So I checked into the hotel and was thrilled when Molly and Holly phoned and asked to meet me at the Joy Cafe down the road. Finally, I'm asked out. I walked there and the port is beautiful; blissfully unaware of the disaster in the hills where 4,500 people were living in garbage bags. (Now there are 8,000.) Tourists stroll, boats bob, the sky blazes blue and around the corner there's mayhem.

I met them at the Joy Cafe and it was indeed joyful because they are my new best friends. Holly has a face like Barbie, framed in long golden hair. (This is the ultimate compliment – I loved Barbie.) Unlike Barbie, she's incredibly smart and has a remarkable personality. I thought she was about eighteen but she must be older because she started saving people seven years ago on the borders of Bosnia where there was no shelter so everyone slept on frozen ground, in the snow-covered forest, watching helplessly as people froze to death. Holly's job was going from person to person to feed those unable to move. They must have thought they'd died and gone to heaven as this beauty queen spoon-fed them. For the next two years, she worked in Serbia and Turkey and other checkpoints as a nurse, all the while searching the web to find volunteers and building up databanks of people who wanted to join in. This is why now she's the main agent for seventy-three camps and supplies a steady stream of 746 volunteers a year. If there's a sudden emergency, she has immediate access to doctors, ditch diggers, engineers, cooks, etc. I asked her how she could do this kind of job. She said she couldn't understand why anyone wouldn't do it. Her mother, she told me, fostered fourteen kids and now tends to people who are dying in her community. Holly said that, when she goes back to London, none of her friends ever ask what she's doing (they don't want to know). I asked her if anything was too much for her and she said there was one thing that still haunts her. She got very close to a pregnant woman at the Bosnian border and even though it was highly dangerous, snuck her and her husband into a hospital to have a scan. They watched the baby moving and her husband was ecstatic because he'd seen his first wife blown up by a bomb. Holly had found out later that the woman tried to escape when she was six months pregnant but, at the border, the guards had kicked the baby out of her.

I thought I'd ask what her philosophy was as she'd clearly become a wise soul from battling the tsunamis of life while I've been lying limp in the jacuzzi. She said she thought our brains are wired to think: *shelter, safety, food.* Once we have those, we don't have anything to worry about and the brain is left with nothing to do and so we create problems, making up things to worry about, and then judge ourselves harshly; worrying about what other people think of us and that we have no value without material success. Working in Samos gives you confidence and makes you feel settled and peaceful.

Her friend and co-worker Molly told me she's the happiest she's ever been. Similar to Holly, in Samos she doesn't feel stress from other people's opinions of her. When she's in London around people who complain about their dissatisfactions, she feels a constant low vibration of stress. 'You pick it up without even noticing and then feel exhausted from them dumping their toxins on you.' Even though these refugees need more than everyone on earth, with not even the basics of food or shelter, here she doesn't feel that low vibration. Here she feels exhilarated. We sat in the Joy Cafe for hours and I loved basking in the heat from their hearts. These girls are the crème de la crème of human empathy and it's catching. The nagging reviewer in my mind finally shut up.

We all went to dinner that night, in a taverna where the owner did a floor show about Pythagoras (father of geometry), who came from Samos and lived in a cave for some reason. The owner performed with such verve, I gave him a standing ovation. Pythagoras, it seems, had a maths cult following like Jim Jones but with equations about triangles, not

Kool-Aid. You'd have to have been a genius to make this interesting but when you're drunk and the performer is equally drunk, it was riveting.

Then Aslam entered, unwashed and smoking, and to my surprise, sat next to me. My sphincter closed. He started to warm up and talk to me because he could see that the girls liked me. He said that he likes to come into this particular place because he can smoke while he's eating and no one minds. He told me he sleeps in coffee shops and calls his computer his girlfriend. I asked him what exactly his role was and it turned out he's a fixer and a great hustler so the refugee charity give him a hunk of money because he knows how to get things done immediately. He has the phone numbers of everyone who can do anything: building playgrounds, opening temporary schools and digging sewers. It ain't one of those big charities like Oxfam or Save the Children, where you have to go through hoops for permits that can take months. This is a feet-on-the-ground charity in its true sense and he is the great mover and shaker behind it, adored by all the volunteers. You don't have to get a hundred famous people singing and dancing to save the world; Aslam, through a haze of smoke, knows how to fix an emergency.

28 March 2019

I can't tell you the joy I felt when I got a message from Aslam telling me to come down to the lobby in ten minutes; he was taking me to the camp. This was like being chosen as High School Prom Queen. When I climbed in the taxi with him, he told me to 'shut up' when I got there, explaining that no one but no one is allowed in the camp unless they're a medical person and I should consider this an honour. So we drove up a cliff, on a zigzag road, which refugees were climbing on foot, carrying plastic tanks of water they'd had to fetch from town. When we arrived, we got out and it was beyond shocking. Thousands of pink and black bin liners blowing in the wind, held down by ropes. Behind each tent were hills of garbage and clotheslines indicating life was still going on. You heard kids laughing as they played kick the can. On our way past the thousands of plastic abodes, a kid around five was carrying two large plastic bottles filled with about forty litres of water each. Aslam tried to help but the kid held on. Then he gave them to Aslam and took my hand, leading me down the hill so I wouldn't slip. His life has come to a dead end, who knows if he has parents, yet he was holding my hand, smiling. When he got to his home, he said to me in English, 'Thank you.' They have to queue for four to five hours for food and if it runs out, savage fights break out for scraps. There is one doctor for 7,000 residents; there is a hospital but the waiting lists are months long. If you do manage to get in, there are no face masks, gloves or much sterilization. When it rains, the whole mountainside of plastic-bag tents gets washed away and they have to build it up again. The camp was equipped for 600 refugees; now there are 7,000. Imagine, these people getting off their rafts after escaping genocide, full of hope and happiness. Then they're picked up by the coastguard, given a plastic sheet to live on or in and are pointed to the mountain. I can't even picture the heartbreak when they realize they've come in for more torture. The local Greeks can't help them because tourism has dwindled, they're broke and there are no jobs; it's a lose-lose situation where everyone is screwed.

On the way back to town, I asked Aslam why someone didn't build toilets and showers. He said he had built a number of portaloos and showers but the Greek mayor of Samos made him tear them down, complaining they were block-ing the road. What road? The real reason was she wanted it to be as deplorable as possible to discourage more refugees from coming. Their other choice is to be massacred at home. I asked how he deals with the local politicians and he told me he's gradually wearing the mayor down. No one else would have the skills of mind-fucking and diplomacy rolled into one. If he does the same job he did on me, she probably assumes she's an idiot by now. Aslam is the only one in charge of distributing resources, not just on Samos but on a number of other islands. Where was the UN or the EU? Not here.

Because of Aslam (now I'm in love . . . again) there are green shoots growing even on this disaster of an island. In a matter of a few weeks, because he sent out smoke signals, there are now pop-up shelters and a newly built women's cen-tre run by (bizarrely) an ex-dancer from Broadway shows like *Chorus Line* and *Cats*. The cafe in the women's centre is pris-tine. I had tea with a beautiful young woman called Princess, with dyed, long, perfectly coiffed purple dreadlocks. Princess told me she uses up all her allocated water to keep her hair clean. She told me her husband was a pop singer in the Congo and wrote a song as a cover for a video showing the police beating up neighbours in the town square. The police came to her house and demanded they hand over the footage. The husband claimed he didn't have it, they didn't believe him and shot her daughter in front of her. Princess was standing in front of me like any young twenty-year-old, wearing an Adidas T-shirt, and the only thing giving away her state was that her legs were shaking, constantly. An Afghan woman told me the authorities took away her eight-year-old son and tortured him for a week, before returning him. He's with her now but so traumatized, he screams all night and never leaves the shack. They're waiting for a therapist who will never come. Last week, her friend in Kabul was kidnapped but her father had no money to pay the ransom, so they hanged her.

I had no idea what to say but wanted to do something rather than just stand there with my mouth hanging open, so I asked if she and her friends wanted me to teach them Pilates and mindfulness the next day. (It's all I've got up my sleeve.) They all said 'yes' without spitting in my face which I would have done to me in their situation.

29 March 2019

They all showed up today; twelve women, some in burkas, saris or designer sportswear. One woman had a shirt on that said in English LIVIN' THE LIFE; hopefully she didn't understand.

So they all got on the yoga mats and I made them do sit-ups while pulling up their pelvic floors. After a few, I asked them if they wanted me to stop because it was too straining for them. They politely said that they were fine. It slowly occurred to me that these women had probably walked through at least six countries with their luggage on their heads and I'm asking if they're tired after ten sit-ups? They could probably do a thousand sit-ups with a grand piano in each hand. Then we did mindfulness and they became calm even though I had horror shows running on a loop tape through my brain.

Later today I took them for manicures. I figured if I was in charge of shallowness, I'd go all the way. Holly and Molly thought it was a great idea. I took them all to a beauty salon, where they spent a great deal of time choosing colours as if it was just a day out with the girls. I have photos of them posing with their new nails. They glowed as they posed like hand models.

Anyway, thrilled with their new (mostly gold glitter) nails, I took them for cappuccinos where we ran into Aslam, who didn't know what expression to put on his face when the women showed him their nails. The women were so humble and dignified as they accepted the coffees and then, without complaint, they departed to walk up a mountain in total darkness. As they walked off, they kept looking at their nails. I hope I did a good thing.

30 March 2019

Aslam gave me a tour of the rest of the island, showing me schools for all ages that he had set up, while Holly had found volunteer teachers through her databank who taught English, maths, IT (Google paid for a tech centre), history, etc.

Aslam was beginning to get my sense of humour, and I got his which was as dark as it comes. He introduced me to his friend from Afghanistan, Imad, who was now a volunteer with the legal team who were helping people get residency to stay in Greece. Imad had escaped and, after a terrifying ordeal, got to Berlin. Miraculously, though he's off-the-chart smart, he got himself into university, studying political science. The details of the terrifying ordeal were that his raft sank halfway across the sea between Turkey and Greece, carrying forty-six refugees including babies. They threw their luggage overboard but when the passengers were up to their knees in water, he and about eight others jumped into the sea and pulled the raft by ropes. When they got to land, he radioed the coastguard for help but they ignored it. Finally, he flagged down some local fishermen to save the half-drowned people and on arrival at Immigration each were thrown a plastic sheet and told to walk up the mountain to the camp. After twenty days in the camp, he escaped, walked to the Macedonian border, slept in the freezing forest and then managed to find a bike which he rode through the mountains in Serbia, finally getting to Hungary where he was thrown into jail and tortured, escaped and got a lift in a truck going to Germany, and that, ladies and gentlemen, is the tale of how he got to Berlin.

He kept a diary and I promised to try and get it to publishers; so far, no publishers have accepted it, even though it's raw and chilling. It's called *The Jasmine Inferno – The Journey of Death*. If there are any publishers out there interested, I have it.

31 March 2019

My last night in Samos and we all went for the last supper. I was trying to make time slow down because I was with people I loved and didn't want to leave them. The cherry on the cake was that Aslam decided to tell me his story. He said he was in Iraq at one point, walking through the desert, when he was given a lift by a helicopter. While it was flying, it was hit by machine-gun fire and they nose-dived. He said he was screaming and vomiting while the guy next to him was shot. Then he stopped and when I pushed him to tell me what happened next, he announced that he was lying, he'd made the whole thing up. See what I mean by a dark sense of humour? I left not knowing anything about him, but I found out no one else did either. He's truly crazy but a hero. I'm still in touch with Holly and Molly and signed up to go back at the end of April 2020.*

* With the coronavirus it will be delayed, but I will go.

My Second World Saver:
GEN (Global Ecovillage Network)

While I was visiting Findhorn (see chapter 1, Community) I met resident and President of GEN-International, Kosha Joubert, who said her vision was to help establish thousands of ecovillages globally from traditional villages in third-world countries through favelas in South America to established or newly built, state-of-the-art communities where people simply wanted low-impact, high-quality lifestyles and an alternative to a culture of consumerism and exploitation.

Kosha said, 'These ecovillages are living laboratories, pioneering alternatives and solutions to enable villages, regions and nations to fulfil the Climate Agreement.' If that's not doing something to save the planet, nothing is. No one planned this community-led movement; instead it emerged from the hearts, minds and hands of courageous people who decided to choose the road less travelled.

The ecovillage movement can be seen as an antidote to the destructive consequences of a dominant world view. The 'market society' simply doesn't work for the vast majority of people: it can never lead to anything but a degraded environment and a disastrous and widening gap between the rich and the poor.

GEN was established in 1995 and so far it's helped create more than 10,000 communities in 100 countries around the world, with some of the lowest recorded carbon footprints per capita. GEN promotes the idea that, 'Every village and city on the planet could become an ecovillage or green city. In a world that is changing faster and faster, we will not be able to react together quickly and effectively without being connected to each other by this web of kinship, the invisible glue that binds us.'

In other parts of the world, governments have taken the model and run with it. For example, in Senegal, GEN helped build a few ecovillages and the Prime Minister was so inspired, he had 14,000 more constructed. He then made a personal commitment to promote ecovillages across the African continent. Kosha says, 'It's time to heal apartheid not in one country but within humanity as a whole.'

Here's How it Works

When they are invited to a prospective community who want to be part of the network, they first listen to the inhabitants' visions of the future and what they'd like to see for their children. Once GEN is sure that the candidate-village's heart is in the right place, they get to work. Depending on each community's diverse needs, they'll help build and train residents to convert to solar energy, use renewable energies, only use regionally sourced materials, to increase biodiversity, practise organic farming, permaculture, water conservation and reforestation. One of their great achievements is that they're using new ways to recycle waste effectively. One day shit, the next day a garden of Eden – that's recycling at its finest.

But what GEN insists on before the first shovel is even lifted is that everyone agrees to its ecological, economic, social and cultural principles. They do, however, ensure that local traditions and rituals remain untouched. The idea is to integrate new innovation with traditional wisdom . . . picture a shaman with an iPhone.

The Five Principles

1. Each member of the community has to work for the well-being of the community by cultivating transparent and

inclusive decision-making. Not judging each other but trying to understand all points of view.

2. The model for decision-making is not a top-down pyramid shape, with a big boss at the top, but a circle where everyone has a say and there's mutual respect. Everyone takes the blame if something goes wrong and reaps the rewards when things go right. GEN teaches various forms of conflict resolution and peace-building skills designed to bring the people closer to true democracy.

3. Gender equality. Imagine the surprise on the faces of men from countries where women are kept in the root cellar (except at feeding and breeding time), when they find out that unless they give women equal power in decision-making, GEN won't be involved. 'Ha ha' is all I can say. GEN's philosophy is that 'every community is only as good as its ability to honour feminine qualities: care, compassion and the ability to listen'.

   GEN also won't tolerate discrimination against any religion or culture – everyone is accepted.

4. Each community has to decide for themselves how land ownership is organized, whether businesses should be run privately or cooperatively, whether the income will be shared or separate and who will look after the members who are ill or elderly. These villages can't be designed by developers, they have to be built by people with a common vision.

5. Each village creates its own economy, but it has to be based on fair trade and ethical systems of exchange. Some use bespoke currencies or Time Banks where you work a certain amount of hours for someone using your particular skills, then they owe you that many

hours working for you. (I like this idea . . . So if I get someone who gardens to do two hours' work then I will probably have to give them two hours of comedy. Also, if they garden well, I'll be funnier, otherwise I'll just crack a few old jokes.)

The Big Deal About GEN

Research on ecovillages concluded that if only 5 per cent of the EU were to engage in effective community-led climate change adaptation initiatives, carbon savings would be sufficient for 85 per cent of its countries to achieve their 2020 emission reduction targets.

Results from Following the Five Principles

- 90 per cent of ecovillages have more than 40 per cent women in decision-making roles
- 90 per cent sequester carbon in soil and biomass
- 96 per cent train in non-violent conflict resolution
- 95 per cent engage in campaigns to protect human rights
- 97 per cent work actively to restore damaged ecosystems in third-world countries affected by floods, drought and other disasters

GEN are also transforming refugee camps into ecovillages through a branch called EmerGENcies, who help coordinate and organize basic needs: food, water, shelter, health and sanitation.

Then there's a NextGEN youth-led global network teaching the next in line to continue the movement of creating and running ecovillages.

✱

I wanted to span the market of ecovillages, to get a taster of what they might have in common. I went to an ecovillage in Cape Town, South Africa, and an ultra-sophisticated one in Ithaca, New York.

Oude Molen, Cape Town

To get there you have to drive down a motorway lined with townships on either side; piles of corrugated tin shanties, which killed me with guilt as I sat in an air-conditioned car drinking a latte.

Oude Molen is located where there was once a prison for murderers. If they were deemed insane after thirty days, they were sent straight to the hospital, do not pass go. If they were diagnosed as not insane, they were in for life, maximum security. From these chilling beginnings, a sustainable little village has sprouted with fifty-five businesses employing 300 people. The guy who started it, John, had to fight the government to stop a development of gargantuan shopping malls (who's going to shop at Zara and have their nails done? Residents from the neighbouring township?). In 1984 when the new government took over, they forgot (on purpose) to budget for these mental hospitals so there were no more resources. John said he'd take care of the people who remained in the hospital and they let him. Good riddance. First of all, he released the patients (brave) and then taught them how to plant seeds and harvest food.

When he first took over, the boys from the nearby townships vandalized the place, stripping it of metal and copper. John caught some of them in the act and, rather than turn them in, asked what their interests in life were. They said, 'Cars,' and he proceeded to teach them about fixing cars – so instead of raiding them, they learnt how to repair them.

There's a very successful mechanical repair service there now and they're making more money than they did by stealing them. In the village populated by 300 people, there's now an internet cafe, a theatre, vegetable stalls, a backpackers' lodge, a school, a medical centre and accommodation for 300 people who come here to do 'shadow' work. (A glorified internship programme, anyone can show up and shadow someone running a business to learn anything from farming to carpentry to coding.)

The nearby township has a million residents with hardly any schooling and zero jobs. This ecovillage is filling the gap; small step by small step but still steps. People wonder why there's so much violence in Africa, throwing up their hands in a 'what do you expect?' gesture. Well, here's your answer – give people somewhere to go to learn a skill along with teaching them regenerative farming and they will come.

Some of GEN's Other International Projects

GEN works in a similar way to B Corp (see chapter 2, Business), giving official accreditation after careful scrutiny to a community that is truly walking the eco talk.

I didn't visit these but they're worth mentioning.

In Favela da Paz, São Paulo, Brazil

Slums take up 24 per cent of Latin America, usually with no electricity, no running water and gang violence 24/7. The garbage hasn't been collected for twenty years.

Jardim Angela favela has 800,000 residents and in the 1990s was ranked by the UNO as one of the most brutal neighbourhoods in the world.

A local guy called Claudio Miranda started playing music

on tin cans. He taught hundreds of street kids to learn the 'tin' and eventually wrote a hit, 'Favela da Paz'. The money came pouring in from everywhere. It was suddenly like 'Favela's Got Talent'. From the funds they built a solar shower which quickly made headline news. From then on he taught the locals how to plant seeds on their roofs to grow food, and now, from an aerial view, you can see green in the favela for the first time. Even more of a miracle, the government has now ordered that the garbage be picked up. Then they joined GEN.

In Kitezh, Russia
GEN helped create an ecovillage dedicated to nurturing foster children who have been abandoned by their parents. Everyone in the community acts as a surrogate family to the kids and gradually, through unconditional love, prepare them to leave when they're emotionally ready to face the real world.

In Sekem, Egypt
Dr Ibrahim Abouleish turned a hot, arid desert into fertile land by building a huge underground irrigation system connected by canals. Once the soil was rejuvenated, farmers from all over Egypt came once a month to learn how to farm without harm and follow the ethos laid down by GEN. He says, 'Economic success is based on brotherliness rather than competition and egoism.' Sekem has opened schools from kindergarten to university for students inside and outside the community. Here they do research in medicine, pharmacy, organic agriculture and economics, and they create new products to adapt to green technologies. Sekem has a medical centre that cares for approximately 40,000 people from surrounding areas.

In Natoun, Togo

This village was in a barren desert where nothing could grow. Menfolk had left the village, unable to deal with the poverty and crying children, leaving the women to fend for themselves. It's now run by a woman who started an initiative, an organic school to teach agriculture, water retention, etc. Once the husbands who left town got wind of how successful the community was, they returned (what a surprise).

In Otepic, Kenya

Similarly, women couldn't speak at the village meetings until one of them piped up and suggested that they made an attempt to enrich the soil. Turns out, she was right, and now 80 per cent of smallholder farmers in the area are women. Someone said (maybe even a man), 'When you reach out to a woman you reach out to an entire village.' Now those women organize women's groups on family planning, AIDs and domestic violence. They also organize peace activities such as football matches between different ethnic tribes and gangs.

As I mentioned, I want to move to an ecovillage. But I think you might know by now, it won't be in a favela or with a tribe but one of the five-star ones. You can't completely change a leopard's spots. Especially mine.

Visiting Ithaca Ecovillage

On 9 July 2019 I went to Ithaca, an ecovillage in upstate New York under the banner of GEN. Again, like at Findhorn, I was expecting a patchouli-oiled, feet-smelling, bean-curd munching hippy commune. A very conservative-looking woman greeted me – almost twinset and pearls – who was

the founder of this twenty-five-year-old intentional community. She developed a new way of rural planning rather than
using the old suburban model which is where a developer
buys a parcel of land and lines the streets with wall-to-wall
homes, to create the most profit. Ithaca ecovillage has no
streets to take up room because you park your car in one of
the two large parking lots just outside the community. (They
also share cars.) The homes face each other, connected by a
squiggly sidewalk with small areas for gardens, playgrounds,
shared bicycles, trampolines, toys and places to mingle in
the middle. The people have the option: they can socialize
out front or, if they want solitude, out the back door they're
facing endless vistas of fields, mountains and lily-padded,
bull-rushed ponds equipped with communal kayaks. Social
in the front, freedom in the back. It's just as financially viable
as any suburban scheme because now that there are fields
available, farmers use them to grow vegetables which they
sell to the city folk of Ithaca, only ten minutes away.

You don't buy your house, you buy shares, and if a building needs repairs and a resident can't afford it, everyone
pitches in to what they call a 'social justice' fund to cover the
cost. If something breaks down in your home or you need
something, you go online and so many volunteers show up
you have to go online again and say, 'Problem solved, don't
come over,' to stop more coming.

Some of the residents told me they moved here because
they wanted to know their neighbours and let their kids run
free. It's multiracial and multigenerational so the elders can
babysit the babies. There is no discrimination against women
or ethnic groups and, if there is, people are asked to think
about departing. It's a mini-mall of writers, software engineers, cleaners, architects, circus performers, professors,
scientists – but they all have to contribute time for two hours

a week towards working for the community: washing dishes, mowing, repairing, administering, whatever your calling is. Everyone has a small allotment for growing fruit and vege- tables and there's even a communally shared cat.

There are three neighbourhoods, Song, Tree and Frog, each differently designed and made of natural stained wood (one looks like a fantasy Western town). Each of the hoods has a gigantic solar panel behind it, providing heating, air conditioning and electricity. Homes have zero net energy and they've generated 13,000 kilowatts in three years, which is equivalent to what a nuclear power plant produces in one day. This is where I may end up living; in a smart home in a smart neighbourhood.

(PS I haven't told my family.)

My Third World Saver: The Kindness Offensive

I heard about this particular movement and was struck by the audacity of the whole idea so I called the founder, David Goodfellow, and found him to be another star in the world- saver stakes. Since he started the Kindness Offensive, he's raised millions of pounds, fed over 5 million people and given away warehouses full of goods to various causes. His story is a jaw-dropper and I don't say that often.

In 2006, his mission began as a way to mitigate his depres- sion. He told me he had spent the last ten years at home, paralysed with fear, feeling as if the walls of his room were a tight-fitting coffin. (Immediately I felt I was with a fellow tribesman.) His childhood friend, Robert, told David about his bizarre hobby; he would cold call various businesses and talk the salespeople on the phone into giving him products for free. He did it by striking up a friendly conversation, making the person laugh and creating a fast-food kind of camaraderie. Basically, he schmoozes them until they break; I call it hustling but David called his friend a 'phone whisperer'. At some point, because David wasn't leaving the house to go anywhere, Robert taught him and some friends the art of phone whispering. He told them when they call to be aware of their facial expressions, posture, tone of voice and attitude, even though they're on the phone. One day, Robert flung a Yellow Pages on the table and told the group to choose a random number. They chose a local Domino's Pizza, Robert did his magic and within thirty minutes they had a free pizza delivered. This guy had a calling to call. After that, David practised tirelessly, mostly getting phones slammed down on him, but on one glorious day a miracle happened and he got the pizza. A successful call can take hundreds of tries and take weeks or months but eventually, like with any great skill, you get the knack; 10,000 hours, you'd be an artist.

Over the years, he and his friends slogged away, filming then critiquing each other. He told me the house started piling up with pots and pans, blenders, a vibrating massage chair, a luxury fish tank and a water-based vacuum cleaner. Word went out about what they were doing and friends and family started to make requests. The hustlers were now being hustled. So far, so self-centred.

A few more years down the line, they got the idea to whisper for strangers and as a social experiment they went into the streets and asked people what they needed, calling it a 'Kindness Offensive'. It held a kind of 'in your face, punk' charm. The next offensive was on 3 August 2008. They set off for Hampstead Heath, asking people, 'How can we help you?' They got eighteen requests, one of them being a guy who said he didn't have any money but wanted to throw a birthday party for his daughter. The next day they 'whispered' to various companies, calling themselves the Kindness Offensive, and a week later they had all eighteen gifts. For the guy with no money, they contacted the Moscow State Circus, who offered not only ringside seats for Chris's daughter's friends but a chance to train with the circus before the show.

Later, a request came from a soup kitchen asking for badly needed food so David and friends somehow ended up whispering to the CEO of one of the largest food producers (they must have been really good by now), who agreed to send twenty-four tonnes of food. None of them knew what that kind of weight meant but pretended to. When the delivery arrived, the football-stadium-sized lorry took up the entire street and, when decanted, the food filled every last crevice in the house so they had to use neighbours' homes. The BBC, hearing about it, turned up and filmed them giving food away to passing strangers, churches, food banks, the Salvation Army and the original soup kitchen, who were now flooded with food. You can imagine, they suddenly got a lot of volunteers. After that they were on a roll, whispering like Olympians; distributing toys and gifts to major hospitals, children's homes, charities and care homes. They received an award from the then Prime Minister for giving the highest number of toys away to kids in hospitals.

David's favourite project was when he got some of his volunteers to go to Trafalgar Square and pretend they needed help after dropping their shopping, falling over or trying to lift a pram upstairs. If a member of the public assisted them, all the volunteers would gather around and sing, 'For He's a Jolly Good Fellow . . .', hand them champagne, flowers, and throw streamers before quickly disappearing, leaving people thinking, 'What the fuck?' I'm sure they'll remember it for the rest of their lives.

I asked David if his people ever use phone whispering to

get something for themselves. He said, 'Actions have consequences; everything you do adds up. If you do evil, well, you
do the math.'

When he gets someone on the phone, he tells them that if
they donate toys, flowers, blankets, food or whatever, the
world will be a better place. The world needs heroes and this
is their chance to be one.

After doing thousands of random acts of kindness, he said
that, 'if you get it right, it affirms the humanity and worthiness of both the giver/performer and the receiver/recipient.
As a performer of the act, you feel worthy and your value is
unquestionable. As the recipient of the act, your worth and
humanity is affirmed by someone giving you a gift without
expecting payback and it's a glimpse into an understanding
that there are kind people in the world, that not everyone is
frightening or out to get you. As someone who suffered
from depression who was haunted by questions like "Am I
good enough? Should I be here?", it offered me an alibi and
purpose.'

My Random Act of Kindness

Just before Christmas I joined David on one of his Random
Acts of Kindness, blitzing the public. We all had to meet in
Camden Town where I was handed a hard hat and neon vest
(their costume) and pointed to a mountain of flower bou-
quets that I was told to load on to the Kindness bus. (He
whispered well to score this particular vehicle.) It's a red
double-decker bus called the Number 42, because Douglas
Adams famously said that 42 is the answer to 'life, the universe and everything'. He wanted the interiors to look like a
1950s American diner; the juxtaposition of a British icon with
a classic American interior. They whispered hard, over a

three-year period, becoming intimate friends/phone bud-
dies with a guy in Germany who had the last remaining
Wurlitzer jukebox in the world. Obviously, in the end he
couldn't say no. Also aboard the bus is a vintage replica
Coca-Cola cooler which you cannot buy in the UK, a gigantic antique gumball machine, two Wesco Spaceboy bins, a
flux capacitor from the *Back to the Future* films (given to them
by George Lucas) and a bar. Aside from all that, there was
nowhere to sit because the bus was packed wall-to-wall with
flowers, toys, boxes of chocolates, cosmetics, perfume,
clothes, sports gear . . . a department store on wheels.

So the bus travels around London, making stops, where
you simply jump off and give a passer-by a gift. At first, I was
a little shy just handing someone random a present and having to explain it was free. We'd both stare at each other as if
it was a joke of some sort while they tried to figure out what
the deal was. I'd have to say a few times, 'No, it's free . . . It's
for you because you're you . . . No, there is no money
involved.' Then I'd see their faces kind of melt into a mile-
wide smile, some people looked in shock or they teared up,
and then I'd jump back on the bus. Well, if you want to get
high on happiness, you can get no better hit than this. I eventually went crazy with rampant *joie de vivre*, chasing people
down the street to hand them the free stuff, just to watch
their eyes as they went childlike on me, like it was their first
Christmas. Once in a while, people brushed my gifts aside or
told me they didn't want anything and I could feel a 'Fuck
you, it's free' swirling up in me. Just as I would catch someone's joy, I'd catch these hardened people's anger and hated
them for it. David advised me to say to myself, 'The recipient
didn't choose to be chosen, it was a random act and I've co-
opted them into a contract that they did not sign up for. Now
I'm upset they aren't paying the debt I forced them into

owing me.' That's why it's best to do this thing as a hit-and-run, don't hang around and expect something back as then it's not an act of kindness.

In my whole life, I don't remember giving something and not expecting something back. Maybe not in concrete terms but there would always be a slight residue of feeling they owed me something later. We blitzed care and children's homes and hospitals that day. Sometimes we'd just leave the gifts at the reception or drop a gift at everyone's door. I never got tired even though it went on for ten hours because I was five years old again and wanted to play. I would do this every day of the week and suggested it, but David can't because it takes him months to whisper for the stuff. I forgot about that part.

At least now I know there's a bus out there somewhere in London that I can get on when I'm low. Imagine if this was a regular service? We should applaud and appreciate all acts of kindness, whoever does them and however they come about. I asked David how he keeps his motives pure. He said, 'I can be an asshole. I can be as thoughtless and polluted as the next guy. I don't go around thinking lofty thoughts and wishing mankind well, but none of that stops me from trying and succeeding to be kind. There is no point in waiting for the pure people to sort everything out. Trust me, they're not coming.

'Life is not a rerun, we don't have stunt doubles or understudies, we're it. The universe doesn't happen to us, we are the universe happening. It actually matters what we do. That's what I'm doing when I phone whisper.'

My Fourth World Saver: Extinction Rebellion – XR

I chose this as a world saver because the people I met at Extinction Rebellion reminded me of who I used to be before

I was dragged into adulthood, kicking and screaming. I recognize the same passion and innocence in their eyes as I had in mine. I had the same spirit to change the world before my lights went out. (They're back on now.) To me, nothing is more energizing than a rebel with a cause. At the few meetings I attended (thinking I totally blended in – totally deluded), in my mind, I was back at Berkeley University, right in the vortex of what was happening; finally, I felt like I was at the right party, at the right time.

I invited one of the founders, Tamsin Omond, over to my house. Juliet Stevenson said we should meet and I obey whatever she tells me to do. Tamsin had brains, wit and beauty; I usually hate people with those qualities but not in this case as she walks the talk. I told her about my riot days and how intoxicating it was to be part of a protest movement. Rebelling was so addictive and in the end I couldn't tell if I was doing it to get a high from the fight, rather than fighting for the cause. I remember being at an anti-war protest at my university and how delicious that adrenaline tasted when caught in the midst of mass madness. I remember going berserk at a policeman, screaming at him that the war was his fault, waving a Vietnamese flag in his face. It turned out he wasn't doing anything, just out taking a stroll. He must have thought I was insane.

The same day, at our first meeting, Tamsin asked me to her wedding and I accepted immediately. It was planned for the first day of the 'International Rebellion', 7 October 2019, on Westminster Bridge at 12.00 p.m. The idea came to her because she wanted to ground the rebellion not in anger but in love. I told her I would dress as the mother of the bride so if I was about to be arrested, I would say I thought I was coming to a wedding; no idea about the rebellion bit. Tamsin has my sense of humour and laughed.

On the big wedding day and first day of the rebellion, I had to fight my way through the throngs of people to where the marriage was to take place. A large mob of us were serenaded by a brass band as we waited for the bride, Melissa MacDonald, to show up. It turned out she was in Parliament Square where her friends had set up a beauty parlour. Her bridesmaids were primping her for her big day; curling her hair, preparing the bouquet and getting her into her wedding dress. Canon Jessica Martin (from Ely Cathedral) married them as helicopters circled above. We sang, threw confetti and cried as Tamsin kissed the bride under the drone of the helicopters.

In the next rebellion, which was supposed to be in May 2020, among other events Tamsin was planning to find fifty people who wanted to get married during the protests so she'd be a kind of XR wedding planner. The couples could choose their location for the wedding anywhere in London, places you could never afford in real life: London Bridge, Trafalgar Square, St Paul's . . . the world would be your oyster. I imagine the police would feel helpless, not wanting to disrupt anyone's Golden Moment. She wanted to call it the Love Rebellion. (Now it really was starting to remind me of the 1960s.)

Even if you think some of the past XR actions may have gone too far and at times pissed off the public, look what they've accomplished in a few short years. They have 1,120 groups in sixty-five countries. The UK alone has over 300 groups. They made visible something that was being ignored by the government and mocked by the press.

I would never have known that each day 100 million tonnes of man-made, heat-trapping global pollution is pumped into our atmosphere, raising the temperature to unprecedented levels. Ninety-three per cent of extra heat is going into the oceans creating storms, each more powerful and destructive than the last. More water vapour is rising from the oceans causing downpours throughout the world, which trigger flooding; eight of them were once-in-a-thousand-year floods in the US in just the last ten years. Also in the last ten years, 1.3 million species representing about 20 per cent of total species have been made extinct. The melting of the Antarctic is causing rising sea levels which may eventually cover Miami, New York, Mumbai; so buy galoshes if you plan to go to any of those. Or if you're planning a holiday in the Maldives, bring a snorkel. So I salute XR in their attempt to focus our awareness on something significant for a change, in a world where we're so easily distracted.

This is their mission and they do what they can through disruption. I asked Tamsin how she cools her engines from battling with a public who either ignore or ridicule the facts of global warming. She does daily meditation, otherwise she finds herself getting too 'grabby' and desperate; falling back into the 'I want, I want' motif, which I know so well. The practice stops her from thinking about what's going to happen tomorrow or in six months (which only whips up the anxiety) and lets her just focus on what's going on now. Also, she says – and I agree – mindfulness helps build up that muscle for compassion like lifting weights at the gym for hard abs. 'The pay-off is when you dole out compassion, it feels good. To be grateful for what you have makes you feel better.'

Using her ability to calm the mind and self-regulate emotions, she trains the XR teams in non-violence and how to stay calm and slow down when things get hectic. 'When you lose your mind, you make mistakes and that's when hot emotions kill the cause.'

Extinction Rebellion follow a code of ethics. (God bless them, it's more than we did back then when our only motto was 'Kill the Pigs'.)

Extinction Rebellion Principles

1. **We have a shared vision of change.** Creating a world that is fit for generations to come.

2. **We set our mission on what is necessary.** Mobilising 3.5 per cent of the population to achieve system change – using ideas such as 'Momentum-driven organising' to achieve this.

3. **We need a regenerative culture.** Creating a culture which is healthy, resilient and adaptable.

4. **We openly challenge ourselves and our toxic system.** Leaving our comfort zones to take action for change.

5. **We value reflecting and learning.** Following a cycle of action, reflection, learning, and planning for more action. Learning from other movements and contexts as well as our own experiences.

6. **We welcome everyone and every part of everyone.** Working actively to create safer and more accessible spaces.

7. **We actively mitigate for power.** Breaking down hierarchies of power for more equitable participation.

8. **We avoid blaming and shaming.** We live in a toxic system, but no one individual is to blame.

9. **We are a non-violent network.** Using non-violent strategy and tactics as the most effective way to bring about change.

10. **We are based on autonomy and decentralisation.** We collectively create the structures we need to challenge power. Anyone who follows these core principles and values can take action in the name of Extinction Rebellion.

I asked Tamsin what past events she loved the most and she said when they pulled a giant pink boat down Oxford Street. She said that rather than more flag waving and raving about the horrors of climate change, this was an act of pure irreverence. You can make people numb by throwing endless facts at them, using words we (mainly me) don't really understand: fracking, greenhouse gas emissions, deforestation, phosphorus loading . . . what do they look like when they happen? I can see Tamsin's point, that in contrast to the almost incomprehensible barking on megaphones, the 'Pink Boat' event was a protest with humour and yet still made a statement about mass consumerism right in the heart of its epicentre, Oxford Circus. One of their principles is not to be self-righteous or worthy like the people who oppose them, who believe in their own rhetoric; that their truth is the real truth and everyone else is deluded. 'Worthiness is the enemy.'

This generation, in general, has far more wisdom than mine did. They realize that an endless craving for more isn't going to make them happy and this taking more than giving back is what's depleting the planet. They've got their eye on the Bigger Picture.

So there you have a close-up snap of four of the most inspiring enterprises I discovered on my journey and, boy, has it been a learning curve.

'All of life is interrelated. We are caught in an inescapable network of mutuality, tied to a single garment of destiny. Whatever affects one directly affects all indirectly' – Martin Luther King Jr

Conclusion

To the Future With Love

I've been writing this book for the last two years, researching and travelling to hunt down wherever the good news
was growing. I feel so privileged I had the chance to see what
humanity looks like when it's at its best; to meet the people
who are planting the seeds for a braver new world. All of
them working towards a less 'I' and more 'we' culture; compassion without borders.

Writing this book has been a kind of treasure hunt, to find
people, places and things that would inspire me to make sub-
stantial changes in my life; that was always my mission. I
knew it was time to maybe cut back on the greed factor but
that's tricky in a world which rewards you for unbridled
greed and ambition. The 'me' generation, of which I'm a
card-carrying member, are so self-obsessed and unaware, we
sucked the planet dry. And lo and behold, just as I was about
to adjust my dials, change my ways and make my amends,
the world juddered to a halt and humanity got the wake-up
call of wake-up calls: Covid-19. Maybe it was nature's way of
telling us that we'd screwed around with it for too long. So
my personal plans have had to be postponed.

The virus still reigns strong, forcing us to stay inside. The
good news is that the air is filled with birdsong which I never
noticed before, maybe because we made too much noise
when we were running the show.

These days I'm running my Frazzled Cafes twice a day on Zoom with 200 people in each session, which gives me a daily snapshot of public opinion. People are in shock, on a roller-coaster ride of emotions because we had no rehearsal for this. In war you can see the incoming coming but this time the enemy could be anyone, anywhere. Some people at the meetings are compulsively busy, exhausting themselves to avoid having to face their thoughts, so they're hoovering like demons or clearing out every cupboard known to man. Others are happy to be doing nothing but then swamped with guilt for feeling okay. Then there are others who, like me, think that this experience is allowing us to push the 'pause' button; giving us time to maybe rethink our lives and figure out what we really want. We've always put that one off (I know I have), telling ourselves we'll figure it out when we retire, when we finally get around to booking that ashram in India, when we make enough money, when we meet that special someone who'll promise to stay with us forever and ever. But happiness was never out there, it is something that springs from the inside; no outside input necessary.

As I said before, writing this book has been a gift; giving me an excuse to meet extraordinary people working in education, community, business, tech and food. What's keeping me from 'going down' during all this is knowing those shoots are still there now and will be there when this is over. I hope I'll be there to join them.

Everyone I met in the book believed that the way we're going to thrive and survive in the future is by working as a team with everyone on the same page rather than striving to win at all costs. The good news is that, against all odds, during this horrendous time, there are even more green shoots sprouting up.

Post Covid-19 Good News

Tech

We used to think communicating screen-to-screen was isolating; now with Zoom, Houseparty, Slack and Amazon
Chime, tech is connecting us in ways I never thought possible. I've noticed on social platforms there's more intimacy,
honesty and vulnerability. Now, especially in my Frazzled
meetings, it's like we're playing tennis with compassion,
returning every ball.

Education

It's a nightmare that kids can't go outside and play, but the
latest online education programmes have come up with
some innovative teaching methods. Already some schools
are moving away from teacher domination to a more collaborative style. Without knowing it, they may be going the
way of Finland.

Business

I'm hoping when this is over we'll not only be cured of the
virus, we'll be cured of the affluenza so many of us have
suffered with. My dream is that we stop worshipping the
corporate 'Masters of the Universe' who only win because
some sucker loses and, instead, reward those who make
the world a better place: teachers, nurses, doctors, care-
takers, delivery people, garbage collectors. And as for those
who, unlike Robin Hood, steal from the poor and give to the
rich, I say, 'Off with their heads!'

Community

If you go on Zoom now, you'll see fine examples of community and compassion; you don't even need to live in a village to feel it, just go online.

World Savers

It's pretty clear that a lot of the things that Extinction Rebellion were wanting changed, changed. An example being the situation in Venice: swans and fish have made an appearance in the now-pristine canals. I'm sure it won't last but right now dolphins are having the time of their lives.

Transformation

Look how quickly we can transform ourselves, almost overnight. We can communicate information and act on it, within minutes. Too bad we didn't stop using plastic bottles as fast as we learnt to hoard loo rolls but, nevertheless, I think we're much humbler now. Compassion also spreads like a virus; last night everyone did a 'clap for the NHS workers' at 8.00 p.m. You could feel the love swooping down the street. I was more connected with my neighbours than in the entire time I've lived here.

My hope is that we remember these feelings of interconnectedness and caring for each other and can possibly keep them going when this is over. This sense of togetherness isn't a new invention. The fact is that everyone and everything really is connected, from the worldwide web of interlinked fungus below the soil to particles in the universe to all the cells in our bodies working as a team to keep us alive.

About 14 billion years ago or thereabouts, a Big Bang

happened, beginning from something microscopic to something doubling in size every trillionth of a second to create the universe. Some elements were dispersed from the explosion, mainly hydrogen and helium, and within three minutes created 98 per cent of all matter that there is or will ever be. Everything, including each of us and the stars above, is more or less made up of these elements. A star could be your cousin. We are all a connected network in this universal lattice of life.

Acknowledgements

Individuals Who've Helped

Researchers: Stephen Buanyi, Camilla More, Joe Dodd
   Publisher: Venetia Butterfield
   Literary agent: Caroline Michel
   PR: Fiona McMorrough, Annabel Robinson
   Copy-editor: Karen Whitlock
   Elizabeth Morrison, director of Frazzled Cafes
   Natasha Gordon, organizer of Frazzled Cafes
   Technology advisor: Peter Read
   Sarajane Aris
   Paul Gilbert
   Margaret Heffernan
   Gelong Thubten, monk
   The whole team at Penguin

Community

Findhorn: Janet Limb
   BedZED: Julia Hawkins, Head of Communication and Policy
   GEN-International: Kosha Joubert

Business

Vincent Stanley, co-founder of Patagonia
   Bart Houlahan of B Corp

Acknowledgements

Tim Munden and Jay Brewer at Unilever
Louise Chester, Mindfulness at Work

Education

REAch2 Tidemill Academy in Deptford, London, and Garden City Academy in Letchworth, Hertfordshire
.b Mindfulness in Schools, Richard Burnett, Chris Cullen and Chris O'Neil
Sir Anthony Seldon, previous head of Wellington College, now Vice-Chancellor of the University of Buckingham
Petter Elo, teacher at Hiidenkivi comprehensive school
Susanna Ahvalo, Kilonpuisto school
Lee Daley at TEDTalks, co-founder of an emerging technology called Hello Genius

Technology

Quantum computing: Hartmut Neven, head of Google quantum department, and Peter Read, tech investor
Headspace: Andy Puddicombe and Richard Pierson
Calm: Michael Acton Smith

Food

John Cherry at Regenerative Farming
Tim Spector, microbe and probiotic expert
Nick Barnard, founder of Rude Health
Miguel Toribio-Mateas, a nutritionist who is also a clinical neuroscientist, specializing in probiotics and mental health

Acknowledgements

World Savers

The Kindness Offensive: David Goodfellow

Samos: Choose Love, Indigo Volunteers, Holly Penalver, Imad Al Suliman, Aslam Obaid and Molly Dignan

Extinction Rebellion: Tamsin Omond and Molly Lipson

Books

Adam Alter: *Irresistible: The Rise of Addictive Technology and the Business of Keeping Us Hooked*

Richard Barrett: *Everything I Have Learned About Values*

Peter Bazalgette: *The Empathy Instinct: How to Create a More Civil Society*

Tal Ben-Shahar: *Happier: Can You Learn to be Happy?*

Alain de Botton: *The School of Life*

Rutger Bregman: *Utopia for Realists and How We Can Get There*

Alex Evans: *The Myth Gap: What Happens When Evidence and Arguments Aren't Enough?*

Nir Eyal: *Indistractable: How to Control Your Attention and Choose your Life*

Paul Gilbert: *The Compassionate Mind*

Yuval Noah Harari: *21 Lessons for the 21st Century*

Johann Hari: *Lost Connections: Why You're Depressed and How to Find Hope*

Rasmus Hougaard and Jacqueline Carter: *The Mind of the Leader: How to Lead Yourself, Your People, and Your Organization for Extraordinary Results*

Meg Jay: *The Defining Decade: Why Your Twenties Matter and How to Make the Most of Them Now*

Acknowledgements

Nathan H. Lents: *Human Errors: A Panorama of Our Glitches, From Pointless Bones to Broken Genes*

Matthew D. Lieberman: *Social: Why Our Brains are Wired to Connect*

Leonard Mlodinow: *Elastic: Unlocking Your Brain's Ability to Embrace Change*

Mark O'Connell: *To Be a Machine: Adventures Among Cyborgs, Utopians, Hackers, and the Futurists Solving the Modest Problem of Death*

Steven Pinker: *Enlightenment Now: The Case for Reason, Science, Humanism, and Progress*

Dr Aric Sigman: *Remotely Controlled: How Television is Damaging Our Lives*

Alex Soojung-Kim Pang: *The Distraction Addiction*

Henry Timms and Jeremy Heimans: *New Power: How It's Changing the 21st Century and Why You Need to Know*

Eric Weiner: *The Geography of Bliss*

Community

Jan Martin Bang: *Ecovillages: A Practical Guide to Sustainable Communities*

Eileen Caddy: *Flight into Freedom and Beyond*

Jonathan Dawson: *Ecovillages: New Frontiers for Sustainability*

Kosha Joubert and Leila Dregger: *Ecovillage: 1001 Ways to Heal the Planet*

Joseph C. Manzella: *Common Purse, Uncommon Future: The Long, Strange Trip of Communes and Other Intentional Communities*

Duncan McLaren and Julian Agyeman: *Sharing Cities: A Case for Truly Smart and Sustainable Cities*

Frederica Miller: *Ecovillages Around the World*

Acknowledgements

Business

Marc Benioff: *Trailblazer: The Power of Business as the Greatest Platform for Change*

Yvon Chouinard: *Let My People Go Surfing: The Education of a Reluctant Businessman*

Yvon Chouinard and Vincent Stanley: *The Responsible Company: What We've Learned from Patagonia's First 40 Years*

Charles Handy: *The Second Curve: Thoughts on Reinventing Society*

Margaret Heffernan: *A Bigger Prize: When No One Wins Unless Everyone Wins*

Frederic Laloux: *Reinventing Organizations*

John Mackey and Raj Sisodia: *Conscious Capitalism*

Kim Polman and Stephen Vasconcellos-Sharpe (eds): *Imaginal Cells: Visions of Transformation*

Alec Ross: *The Industries of the Future*

Douglas Rushkoff: *Team Human*

Raj Sisodia and Michael J. Gelb: *The Healing Organization: Awakening the Conscience of Business to Help Save the World*

Raj Sisodia, David B. Wolfe and Jag Sheth: *Firms of Endearment: How World-Class Companies Profit from Passion and Purpose*

Education

.b: *An Introduction to Mindfulness in Schools*

Alex Beard: *Natural Born Learners: Our Incredible Capacity to Learn and How We Can Harness It*

Sir Ken Robinson: *Creative Schools: Revolutionizing Education from the Ground Up*

Anthony Seldon: *The Fourth Education Revolution: Will Artificial Intelligence Liberate or Infantilise Humanity*

Acknowledgements

Food

Louise Foxcroft: *Calories and Corsets: A History of Dieting Over 2,000 Years*

Tim Spector: *Spoon-Fed: Why Almost Everything We've Been Told About Food is Wrong*

Bee Wilson: *First Bite: How We Learn to Eat*

World Savers

Piero Ferrucci: *The Power of Kindness: The Unexpected Benefits of Leading a Compassionate Life*

Nora Gallagher and Lisa Myers: *Tools for Grassroots Activists: Best Practices for Success in the Environmental Movement*

Paul Hawken: *Drawdown: The Most Comprehensive Plan Ever Proposed to Reverse Global Warming*

Professor Michael Puett and Christine Gross-Loh: *The Path: A New Way to Think About Everything*

Index

Abouleish, Ibrahim 210
Adams, Douglas 216
addiction, to technology 134–6, 154–5
advertising 133
Agyeman, Julian 24
Ahvalo, Susanna 119–22
Air-Ink 143
Anderson, Alexander P. 165
Andhra Pradesh 178
Anglian Water 36–7
animals 48–50
Aoun, Joseph 147
Appert, Nicolas 161
Aristotle 90
Atkins Diet 168, 173
Aunt Jemima pancakes 163–4

B Corp 66–70, 209
bacteria 173–6, 182–3
banks 42, 45, 52
Banting, William 168, 169, 171
Barnard, Nick 163
Beard, Alex 85, 113
BedZED eco-community 27–8
bees 142
Ben & Jerry's 71, 74
Beverly Hills Diet 169
Bezos, Jeff 39
Big Bang 228–9
bio-couture 139
Bowen, Joanna 21–2, 33, 36, 164
brains
    and body parts 129
    deep brain stimulation 138
    linking 15

Brazil 209–210
bread 164
Breatharian Diet 170
Brooke Bond 74
Buddha 171
business 38
    B Corp 66–70
    and community 36–7
    conscious capitalism 56–9
    green shoots 51–3
    greenwashing 54
    history of 42–6
    Patagonia 59–66
    post Covid-19 good news 227
    reasons for change 53–6
    Ruby's story 40, 55–6
    and status 46–7
    Unilever 70–79
    where we are now 38–42

Caddy, Eileen 30–32, 33, 36
Caddy, Peter 30–31, 32
Callas, Maria 162
Cape Town 208–9
capitalism 41, 44
    conscious capitalism 56–9
    see also business
carbon dioxide (CO_2) 55, 181
cassava 141
cereals 164–5, 180
Chen, Marc Collins 27
Cherry, John 181, 182
Chester, Louise 75–7
Chicago Democratic Convention
    185–8

237

China 123
  death by work 39
  education 95–102, 110
Chouinard, Yvon 59, 61–2, 64
Churchill, Winston 48
cities 23–5
  BedZED eco-community 27–8
  floating 27
  living cities 25–6
  non-tech solutions 26
cleverness 85
climate change 64, 71, 123, 181, 220–21
Clouds Over Sidra 150
Cognitive Behavioural Therapy
  (CBT) 147–8
comedians 13–14
community 10, 18
  connection 12–14
  Frazzled Cafes 17–18
  in future 22–37
  linking brains 15
  loneliness 11–13
  post Covid-19 good news 228
  Ruby's story 14–17, 19–22, 34–5
Community Markets for
  Conservation (COMACO) 178
compassion 8–9, 156, 221, 225, 228
computers
  mindfulness exercises 155–6
  quantum computing 143–4
conscious capitalism 56–9
  B Corp 66–70
  Patagonia 59–66
  Unilever 70–79
Conscious Capitalism (Mackey and
  Sisodia) 57–8
consumption 47
Copenhagen 24–5
corporations *see* business
Coursera 104
Covid-19 ix, 225–6, 228
  homeschooling 94
  lockdown 12
  post Covid-19 good news 227–8

Crisco 167
Crispr 5
Crystals of Kaydor 149
cycling 25

Daley, Lee 105
Daley, Richard 186–7, 188
Darcy, Alison 147
Darwin, Charles 47–8, 49
Davidson, Richard 148–9
Dawkins, Richard 50
deep brain stimulation 138
desalination 142
Dickens, Charles 79
The Diet Myth (Spector) 175
diets 168–73
Dirt (Montgomery) 159
Domestos 74
Dove 75
Dunbar, Robin 12
Dynasties 49

early learning 85–6, 102–3
eco-communities 27–8
Ecological Intelligence (Goleman)
  138–9, 183–4
ecovillages 28–30
  Findhorn 30–36
  GEN 36, 204–213
edible packaging 142
edible spoons 142
education
  in China 95–102
  early learning 85–8, 102–3
  in Finland 113–22
  history of 88–93
  importance of failure 82
  league tables 94–5
  measuring success 113
  post Covid-19 good news 227
  REAch2 106–113
  rethinking 80
  Ruby's story 81, 83–4
  smartness 85

Index

and technology 102–6
what's not working 84
where we are today 93–4
Egypt 210
Einstein, Albert 9, 113
Elo, Petter 116, 117
EmerGENcies 207
emotional intelligence, and
    technology 147–54
empathy training 149, 150–51
environment 55
    climate change 64, 71, 123, 181,
    220–21
    sustainable innovations 138–43
EOSTA 178
evangelical churches 14–15
Extinction Rebellion 218–22,
    223, 228
    principles 222–3

Facebook 131–3, 135, 136
failure 82, 83–4
farmers markets 178–9, 180
farming 159, 180–81
    COMACO 178
    food waste 179–80
    Regenerative Agriculture 182
    Zero Budget Natural
        Farming 178
fasting 170–71
fats 167, 168–9
Favela da Paz, São Paolo 209–210
fear 3, 145
Feedback 179
Findhorn Community 30–36, 204
Finland, education 113–22, 227
5:2 diet 170
floating cities 27
food 157–8
    cereals 164–5
    diets 168–73
    farming 180–82
    fats 167, 168–9
    good news for the future 176–9

history of 158–65
humans and plants 182–4
probiotics 173–6
Ruby's story 163–4, 170
sugar 165–6
vegetarianism/veganism 171–2
waste 179–80
Franklin, Benjamin 161
Frazzled Cafes 17–18, 226, 227
Friedman, Milton 44, 50
Fuld, Richard 45–6
fungi 139–40, 183
future 1
    fear of 5–6
    and hope 9–10
    Ruby's story 1–2
Futurelearn 104

Gandhi 171
garbage see waste
Garbo, Greta 15
Garden City Academy,
    Letchworth 106, 107–113
Gehl, Jan 24
GEN (Global Ecovillage Network)
    36, 204–5
    five principles 205–8
    Ithaca ecovillage 208, 211–13
    other international projects
    209–211
    Oude Molen 208–9
Generation Y see millennials
Gilbert, Paul 9
Gleaning Network 179
global warming 64, 71, 123, 181,
    220–21
Goleman, Daniel 76, 138–9, 183–4
Goodall, Jane 49
Goodfellow, David 213–18
Google 60
Grant, Adam 113
greed 45, 47–8, 52, 225
greenwashing 54
gut bacteria 173–6

Index

Harari, Yuval Noah 146
Hayek, Friedrich 50
health
    and food 157, 158, 165–6, 167
    work-related deaths 39
hedge fund managers 51
Hello Genius 105–6
Helsinki 114–15
Hilton, Paris 12
Hitler, Adolf 3
Houlahan, Bart 67–8
Human to Human 153–4
Humphrey, Hubert 187

Impact Hub Brixton 177
India 178
Indigo Volunteers 189
Industrial Revolution 43, 91–2
inequality 39, 41, 71, 123
Instagram 132
intentional communities see
    ecovillages
isolation see loneliness
Ithaca ecovillage 208, 211–13

Jackson, Michael 170
James, William 85
Japan
    death by work 39
    education 95
    Paro 152
Jardim Angela favela, São Paolo
    209–210
The Jetsons 1
Jews
    ice 161
    money 43, 45
Joseph and the Amazing Technicolor
    Dreamcoat 161
Joubert, Kosha 204, 205

Kenya 211
ketosis 171
Keynes, Maynard 128

Keys, Ancel 168
The Kindness Offensive 213–18
King, Martin Luther, Jr 223
Kitezh, Russia 210
KOMP 152
Korea, suicide rate 98
Krieger, Mike 132
Kuma, Kengo 25–6
Kurzweil, Ray 129, 130

Laloux, Frederic 52–3, 56
league tables 94–5
Lebow, Victor 47
Lee, Suzanne 139
Lehman Brothers 45–6
Leo, Pope 43
Let My People Go Surfing
    (Chouinard) 59
Letchworth Garden City Academy
    106, 107–113
Lever, William 72–3
life expectancy 7
Lifebuoy 74
lighting 141–2
Liter of Light 141–2
literacy 7
'The Little Mermaid' 121–2
living cities 25–6
London, BedZED eco-community
    27–8
London Grows 177
loneliness 11–13, 26
    and robots 151–2
Lucas, George 217
Luther, Martin 90–91

McCallum, Ian 52
McCarthy, Gene 185, 187
MacDonald, Melissa 220
Mackey, John 57
McLaren, Duncan 24
Maclean, Dorothy 31
Martin, Canon Jessica 220
Massachusetts 91

Mazel, Judy 169
Me: A Kid's Diary 150
Mead, Margaret 156
medicine, and technology 137–8
mental health, innovative
    technology 145–56
microbes 173–6, 182–3
millennials, and business 53–6, 64
mindfulness 7–8, 34, 221
  and business 75–9
  in schools 95, 106–113
  and technology 145–6, 154–6
Minnelli, Liza 169
Miranda, Claudio 209–210
mission 58
Miyako, Eijiro 142
mobile phones 126
  mindfulness exercises 155–6
Montgomery, David 159
Munden, Tim 72, 73
mycelium 139–40

Napoleon 161
Natoun, Togo 211
Natural Born Learners (Beard) 85, 113
Nea Kavala refugee camp 189–95
Neoliberalism 45
Netflix 136
Netherlands 178
neural connections 15
Neven, Hartmut 143–4
New York, garbage collectors 47
NextGEN 207
No Isolation 151–2
Nørrebro, Copenhagen 24–5

Ocean Cleanup 143
Oceanix City 27
Omega Point 130
Omond, Tamsin 219, 220, 221, 223
On the Origin of Species (Darwin)
  47–8
online courses 103–5, 227
Oodi Helsinki Library 114–15

Orchard Project 178
Otepic, Kenya 211
Oude Molen, Cape Town 208–9
oxytocin 13, 14

Paleo Diet 171
Paro 152
Patagonia 59–66
Peabody Trust 27–8
peace 7, 48
Pearlman, Leah 132
People's Fridge 177
pet alternatives 152
PG Tips 74
phone whispering 213–17
PISA (Programme for
  International Student
  Assessment) 95
plastic 140
  alternatives to 140–41
Plato 90, 124
Poleman, Paul 70–71, 72
Pollan, Michael 172
Port Sunlight 72–3
poverty 7, 50
Prakash, Manu 138
Presley, Elvis 169
probiotics 173–6
puffed rice 165
purpose 56–8, 70, 71–2, 74–5

quantum computing 143–4

Random Acts of Kindness 213–18
Random App of Kindness (RAKi)
  150–51
Ranpura, Ash 22
REAch2 106–113
Reagan, Ronald 44
refugees 188–9
  EmerGENcies 207
  Nea Kavala refugee camp 189–95
  Samos refugee camp 195–203
Regenerative Agriculture 182

Index

Reinventing Organizations (Laloux)
    52–3, 56
Rickman, Alan 83
Robinson, Ken 105
robots 6, 123, 126, 129
    jobs that can't be replaced by 128
    jobs that will be replaced by 127–8
    and loneliness 151–2
Rosenstein, Justin 132
Rothschild, Mayer Amschel 43
rubbish *see* waste
Russia 210

Saltwater Brewery 142
Samos refugee camp 195–203
Sanders, Colonel 162
São Paolo 209–210
Seabin Project 142
seaweed 140–41
Sekem, Egypt 210
Seldon, Sir Anthony 95–6
self-help 4–7
The Selfish Gene (Dawkins) 50
Senegal 205
Shanghai 95–102
sharing 24
Sharing Cities (Agyeman and
    McLaren) 24
Shaw, Bernard 56–7, 171
Shelley, Percy Bysshe 171
Singapore
    education 95
    living cities 25
The Singularity is Near
    (Kurzweil) 130
Sisodia, Raj 57–8
Sleeping Beauty Diet 169–70
smartness 85
Snapchat 132
Socrates 90, 116, 123–4
South Africa, Oude Molen 208–9
Spector, Tim 172, 173, 174, 175
Spencer, Herbert 50
SpinCycle 142–3

Stanley, Vincent 60, 61–6
status 46–7
Stevenson, Juliet 83, 189, 219
Strasburger, Vic 102–3
sugar 165–6
summer camp 19–20
survival of the fittest 47–8, 50
Sydney, Seabin Project 142

technology 123–4
    addiction to 134–6
    advertising and data hacking
        133, 136
    the bad news 126–31
    and business transparency 63
    and education 102–6
    fear of 123, 130–31
    for good 136–54
    history of 124–6
    in medicine 137–8
    for mental health 145–56
    mindfulness exercises 154–6
    post Covid-19 good news 227
    quantum computing 143–4
    Ruby's story 126
    sustainable innovations 138–43
    where it might have gone
        wrong 131–3
Thatcher, Margaret 44, 50, 93
Thoreau, Henry 13
Thubten 21, 22
Tidemill Academy, Deptford 106
Time Banks 205–6
Togo 211
Tokyo 25–6
Toribio-Mateas, Miguel 174–5, 176
trans fats 167
transformation 228–9
transhumanists 130
Trump, President 3, 45, 62, 123, 131

Udemy 104
'The Ugly Duckling' 122
UN Habitat 27

Index

Unilever 70–79
United States
  business 39, 40, 53, 68
  Chicago Democratic
    Convention 185–8
  education 91
  farmers markets 179
  food 157, 162–4, 167
  heart disease 158
  Ithaca ecovillage 208, 211–13
urban planning 23–8
urge surfing 155

veganism 171–2, 173
vegetarianism 171–2
Venice 228
video games 148–51
virtual reality (VR) 150
vision 58

Wall Street 45
war 48, 50, 160–61
waste 157–8
  food 179–80
  GEN ecovillages 205
water, desalination 142

Waterlily 142
Watson, Julia 26
Watt, James 129
Wellington College, Shanghai 95,
  99, 100–102
Wisbech 36–7
Woebot 147–8
women
  in business 62, 73
  GEN ecovillages 205
  self-help 4
world savers 185, 188, 223
  Extinction Rebellion 218–23
  GEN 204–213
  post Covid-19 good news 228
  Ruby's story 185–8
  Samos refugee camp 188–203
  The Kindness Offensive 213–18

XR see Extinction Rebellion

Yunus, Muhammad 51–2

Zambia 178
Zero Budget Natural Farming 178
Zuckerberg, Mark 131–3, 134–5, 136